SUCCESSFUL
WEIGHT LOSS WITH
THE GASTRIC
SLEEVE

Guillermo Alvarez, M.D.

ISBN: 978-1502464613

www.thegastricsleeve.com

Printed and bound in the United States of America

Published by MBM Publishing
4000 East Bristol Street, Suite 3
Elkhart, IN 46514

Dedication

To my parents, for giving me education
and non-stop support throughout my
life; to my staff, for helping me change
people's lives in so many ways every
day, without them I am nobody; and to
my patients, for the enormous support,
education, and a shared passion for
bariatric surgery.

About this Book

This book will help you understand in depth the gastric sleeve procedure, also known as sleeve gastrectomy. It will guide and help you through the weeks, months and even years ahead. There is a lot of information contained, so we ask that you please read through everything carefully since many of your questions will be answered here.

Remember, this is only a guide and your mileage may vary.

I am giving you the basic tools to be as successful as you can be. The rest is up to you. Compliance is the key to your success and well-being. If you have any questions we suggest you contact your doctor's office or you can contact me via my website www.endobariatric.com.

I also suggest you join a support group physically or virtually. There are a lot of people out there who have been "sleeved," and not feeling alone in this world helps a bunch. There are several weight loss surgery online communities out there that can help you meet other people and share experiences.

Also you can join my gastric sleeve support group on Facebook by searching Endobariatric.com in the search box. In this Facebook group you'll have the opportunity to meet and talk to many of my patients. Come in and join the conversation.

Finally, you can follow me on Twitter as well (**@endobariatric**) or like my fan page on Facebook (**www.facebook.com/endobariatric**) for updated info on the weight loss surgery world, specifically on the gastric sleeve.

Best of luck on this journey!

Guillermo Alvarez, M.D.

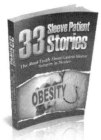

Get a FREE Copy of 33 Gastric Sleeve Stories From My Patient Files

Go to www.SleeveStories.com

Disclaimer

The objective of this book is to acquaint you with the gastric sleeve or sleeve gastrectomy procedure. The information, services, products, messages, and other materials contained here are provided for educational and general information purposes only and are not a substitute for medical advice and treatment. The inclusion of medical information is not intended to create a caregiver-patient relationship. The answers are for informational purposes only and they do not imply diagnosis or treatment and should always be used in conjunction with the advice of your personal health care provider. Any representation contained here is not intended to expressly or implicitly warrant or create any standard of care. Once again, it is not intended to replace medical advice from your health care provider.

Table of Contents

Chapter 1

What is Obesity?

Obesity is defined by The American Obesity Association as the excessive accumulation of adipose tissue to an extent that health is impaired.

Obesity in an adult is determined by using weight and height to calculate a number called the "body mass index"(BMI). The reason the BMI is used is that, for most people, it correlates with their amount of body fat and is related to the risk of disease and death. The score is valid for both men and women. Body Mass Index or BMI is a number calculated from a person's weight and height. The BMI provides a reliable indicator of body fatness for most people and is used to screen for weight categories that may lead to health problems. There are several online calculators you can use to determine your BMI. Official websites like the Center for Disease Control and Prevention (www.cdc.gov) or the U.S. Department of Health and

Human Services with the National Heart, Lung and Blood Institute (www.nhlbi.nih.gov) have trustable body mass index calculators.

The International Classification of adult underweight, overweight, and obesity according to BMI.

	Obesity Classification	BMI Range
Underweight		<18.5
Normal		18.5 – 24.9
Overweight		24.9-29.9
Obese	I	30-34.9
Obese	II	35-39.9
Morbidly Obese	III	>40

The obesity epidemic has come to our attention and is a growing and severe problem to assess. With globalization, our lifestyles, with lack of exercise and other factors, have become some of the major issues that contribute to this epidemic. This problem has not only become an issue in the United States of America, but is becoming a worldwide epidemic. In America, the Center for Disease Control (CDC) in Atlanta, Georgia, has described society as "obesogenic" due to the tendency of being obese due to non-healthful foods, increased food intake, and the lack of physical activity. The World Health Organization has called it "globesity." Obesity is one of the leading preventable causes of death worldwide. The lowest mortality risk has been found in people with a body mass index between 20 and 25. The higher your BMI, the higher risk of death you have. A BMI above 32 has been associated with a doubled mortality rate among women. In the United States obesity is estimated to cause 111,909 to 365,000 deaths per year, while 1 million (7.7%) of deaths in Europe are attributed to excess weight. On average, obesity reduces life expectancy by six to seven years, a BMI of 30-35 reduces life expectancy by two to four years, while morbid obesity (BMI > 40) reduces life expectancy by ten years.

Chapter 2

Treatment Options for Weight Loss

Non-surgical treatment options for weight loss

Exercise and diet

This option is the most used line of treatment for obesity. The idea is to limit the amount of caloric intake and increase the energy expended. Unfortunately, it has not proven to be a good option for the morbidly obese since it does not give good results in these patients. In these patients in particular, the diet and exercise work while they stay with them. However, once the patient stops dieting and/or exercising, the weight usually comes back on, often with extra pounds.

Pharmacotherapy

Medications also play a role in the treatment of obesity. Although everyone cannot use medications, they are usually prescribed for patients with a BMI of ≤30 or a BMI of ≥27 if concomitant obesity-related risk factors or diseases exist (e.g. high blood pressure, diabetes, etc.). These medications have side effects that usually include increase in blood pressure, tachycardia (elevated heart rate),reduction in the absorption of fat-soluble vitamins and other nutrients, and other side effects. The FDA has approved some medications for long-term use, but these medications will only help while the patients are taking them. Again, with this method the weight usually comes back after finishing or abandoning the treatment, and not all patients respond to a given drug.

Over-the-counter medications are usually medications sold in drugstores and don't require a prescription. There are hundreds of medications out there that fit in this category; most haven't been proven safe and effective, and some can even jeopardize your health. Most of these medications or supplements aren't subject to the same rigorous standards as are prescription drugs.

Due to the disadvantages of many of these treatments, patients often seek a more reliable approach to their weight problems. Surgery may provide an option for these people.

Surgical options for weight loss

Bariatric surgery has been around since the 1950s. Bariatric surgery is also known as weight loss surgery or obesity surgery and is widely accepted as the only known effective treatment for severe obesity. As we will discuss, there are other options for weight loss, such as low-calorie diets and exercise, but these have proven to fail or have limited success on long term follow-ups in morbidly obese patients, and surgery is currently the best-established and most successful method for sustained weight loss in these patients. Also, it has been shown to improve or resolve other conditions related to obesity like type II diabetes, hypertension, and sleep apnea, among other conditions. Obesity surgery can offer the patient a better quality of life and improve chances of an enhanced life span.

Weight loss surgeries can be divided into three main categories: First we have the restrictive surgeries, which are procedures that limit the amount of food a patient can eat at a time. Second there are the malabsorption procedures, which are surgeries that reroute food through the digestive tract so the body is able to absorb only a fraction of the nutrients food can supply. The third category is a combination of the first two, providing both a restricted intake and poor calorific absorption. I will explain the following procedures, which are the most common weight loss surgeries within each category.

Vertical Banded Gastroplasty

The vertical banded gastroplasty (VBG) is a restrictive procedure rarely done nowadays because of very poor weight loss and high percentage of long-term complications compared to other weight loss procedures. It consists of creating a gastric pouch based on the lesser curvature of the stomach created by a stapler device. The outlet of this pouch is restricted with a prosthetic band or mesh. The VBG is a purely restrictive procedure.

This procedure used to be very popular because it is a simple operation and has a low risk of early surgical complications.

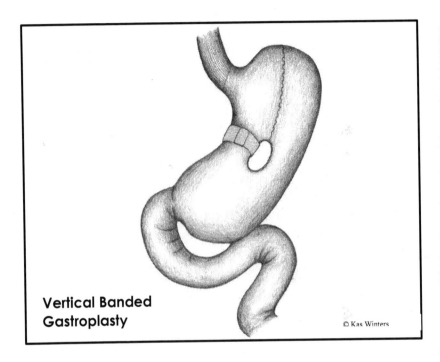

Vertical Banded Gastroplasty

© Kas Winters

Although short-term results looked promising, long-term results were not favorable and were associated with complications and this procedure has practically been abandoned.

Laparoscopic Adjustable Gastric Banding

The adjustable gastric band is a reversible restrictive procedure done through laparoscopy (also known as "key hole" or minimal invasive surgery). Recovery from this surgery is rapid, and patients are managed as outpatients or spend one night in the hospital. The procedure was very attractive when it was approved by the FDA in 2001 since it is done through minimal invasive surgery, it is adjustable, and it is reversible. But when it comes to results (long term weight loss), costs for fills (maintenance) and the quality of life for patients (vomiting, gastro esophageal reflux, restriction on certain foods like bread, meat, etc.) it has been losing popularity. The two FDA-approved bands are LAP-BAND®, from Allergan, based in Irvine, California, and the Realize® band from Ethicon Endosurgery in Cincinnati, Ohio. These bands are made of silicone and have an inflatable ring on the inner surface that can be filled with saline to a desired amount to limit the amount of food a patient can intake at a time. The adjustments or fills are done starting approximately week 4-6 and then at 2-to 3-month intervals until the optimal level is achieved. These fills are done as an outpatient procedure in the surgeon's office either with or without the use of X-rays or a fluoroscopy machine. Being a foreign body inside, patients normally develop complications like band slippage (displacement), band erosion and/ or port –site infections finally leading the patient back to the operating room for the removal of the band and possibly regaining some of the weight he/she had lost.

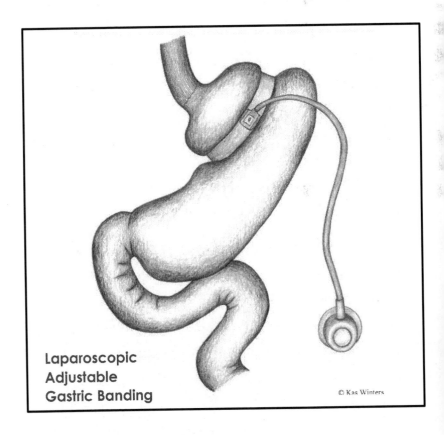

Laparoscopic
Adjustable
Gastric Banding

© Kas Winters

Gastric Plication

The Gastric Plication is a new approach and is another option as a restrictive bariatric procedure. The term plication refers to the rounded shape of the stomach made by folding it in layers. Short term results seemed to show similar results as the Gastric Bypass or the Gastric Sleeve but long term results are not as promising with weight regain and unsuccessful weight loss. It was a procedure that looked promising at the beginning being a short surgical procedure, not involve cutting or stapling of the stomach which made surgeons think that it probably eliminated the risk of a leak, which is the most feared complication of a Gastric Bypass, Gastric Sleeve. The first part of the procedure is done in a very similar way as the Gastric Sleeve where the greater curvature of the stomach is separated from the vessels, and greater omentum which is a large fatty structure in the abdomen that drapes over the intestines like an apron. After this is done, normally a 32 Fr calibration tube, or bougie, is then placed to perform the plication or folding of the stomach. At this point, a first layer of non-absorbable interrupted stitches is placed, followed with two more layers of non- absorbable running sutures to form the plication in form of a sleeve. A major disadvantage of the Gastric Plication is that no long- term studies exist; therefore, the long-term results are unknown. Also, reversibility or conversion to another weight loss surgery is questionable. Very few ongoing clinical trials are currently studying this procedure up-close and the procedure is still considered "experimental" and not approved by the American Society for Metabolic & Bariatric Surgery (ASMBS).

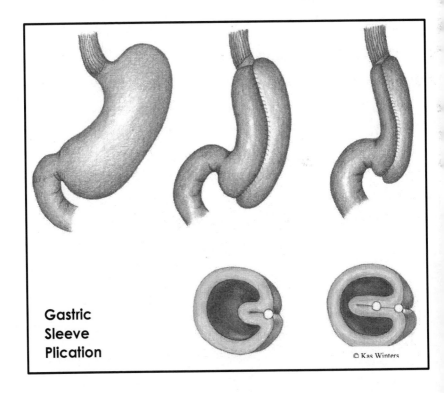

Gastric Sleeve Plication

© Kas Winters

Roux-en-Y Gastric Bypass

The gastric bypass is an operation that combines both restriction and mal-absorptive components. In other words, it is designed to limit the amount you are able to intake because the stomach is reduced greatly to a small pouch, and, in addition, your intestines are re-routed to intentionally make you not absorb the nutrients/calories of the food you intake. Today, the most popular version of this gastric bypass is done laparoscopically with tiny incisions, which gives the patient the benefit of a rapid recovery. The traditional open version of surgery is still done, but it is mostly reserved for difficult scenarios, for example a patient with previous abdominal or weight loss surgery, very

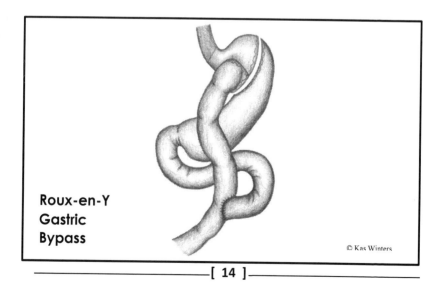

Roux-en-Y
Gastric
Bypass

© Kas Winters

high BMI patients, or when the surgeon does not feel comfortable with the laparoscopic technique. The operative time is generally between 2 to 4 hours. This procedure is considered safe and a very effective operation but has some disadvantages that we will discuss further in a later section.

Biliopancreatic Diversion and Duodenal Switch

The biliopancreatic diversion (BPD) was developed by Professor Nicola Scopinaro in the late 1970s. It is a drastic mal- absorptive operation carried out by re-routing intestines, but also has a restrictive component accomplished by partially cutting out the stomach (subtotal gastrectomy), leaving a 10-15 oz gastric pouch. This operation is very complex and technically more challenging than any of the surgeries mentioned previously. The duodenal switch is a modification of the BPD, but instead of doing a subtotal gastrectomy, a gastric sleeve is performed having greater restriction. There are also some other minor differences in these procedures, but mentioning them would go beyond the objectives of this book.

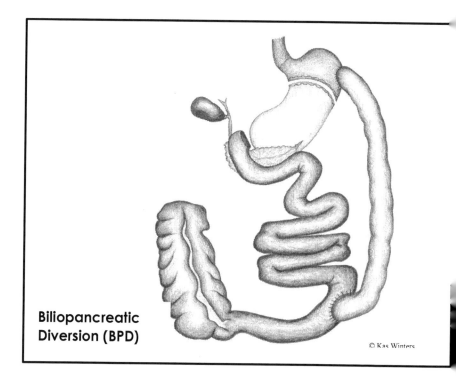

Biliopancreatic Diversion (BPD)

© Kas Winters

The Gastric Sleeve or Sleeve Gastrectomy

The gastric sleeve has recently become an increasingly common and popular restrictive operation. This is a restrictive surgical weight loss procedure that will limit the amount of food you can eat and will help you feel full sooner. The procedure originated as part of a duodenal switch operation and later evolved into a staging procedure for super obese or high-risk patients.

The postoperative course is similar to a gastric bypass. Typically, an upper gastrointestinal study is performed 24 hours after the surgery to evaluate the absence of a leak from the staple line. After this, patients can be discharged on the first or second postoperative day, depending on the surgeon's preference. We will talk more about this procedure in the following sections.

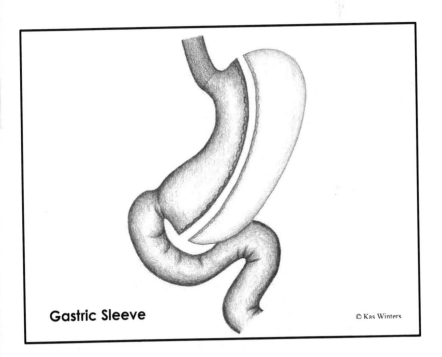

Gastric Sleeve

© Kas Winters

Chapter 3

The Gastric Sleeve: What is the Procedure?

The Gastric Sleeve (GS) is a restrictive surgical procedure done through laparoscopy, (minimal invasive surgery) also known as "keyhole surgery," in which a percentage of the stomach is taken out.

Depending on the surgeon, this resection maybe between 60% to 80% of the stomach.

The remainder of the stomach that is left in place will carry out all the functions (digestive, acid secretion, etc.) perfectly well for the rest of the patient's life. This will work out as a restrictive procedure limiting the amount of food the patient intakes. This procedure does not involve altering (re-routing) intestines at all like in the gastric bypass; therefore, issues of vitamin deficiencies are rarely seen with the gastric sleeve since the stomach will digest the food and the intestine will absorb 100% of the nutrients. It is also it is a much simpler operation to do and carries less risk as well. On average, the surgery time is 35 minutes for a gastric sleeve surgery. This short OR time is transmitted to the patient as improved safety. With less time in the OR and less time under anesthesia, the percentages of possible complications in the OR are reduced. Differences between the gastric sleeve and other weight loss procedures will be discussed also.

The Gastric Sleeve procedure goes by other names:

- Vertical Sleeve Gastrectomy
- Sleeve Gastrectomy
- Vertical Gastrectomy
- Vertical Gastroplasty
- Greater Curvature Gastrectomy
- Parietal Gastrectomy
- Gastric Reduction
- Longitudinal Gastrectomy

History of the gastric sleeve

The gastric sleeve is an evolution of previous procedures that originated since 1987, but the concept of the gastric sleeve is similar to a modified restrictive procedure called the Magenstrasse and Mill procedure (M & M). A group in Leeds, United Kingdom, first described this surgery in 1995. The name M & M comes from "Magenstrasse" referring to the new long narrow channel created and "Mill" referring to the grinding of the food bolus that is carried out in the area before it passes to the duodenum. This procedure creates several gastrointestinal problems like dumping syndrome (food moves into the small intestine quickly and is mostly undigested), diarrhea, nausea, and vomiting, and was abandoned as a weight loss procedure. The gastric sleeve was first performed by laparoscopy (keyhole surgery) by Dr. Michel Gagner at the Mount Sinai Hospital in New York City in 1999. A year later, Gagner proposed the gastric sleeve be the first step of a two-stage duodenal switch on a high-risk group. Then, in 2003, the procedure was proposed as a first step of a two-stage Roux-en-Y gastric bypass. Since then the gastric sleeve has gained popularity and acceptance by surgeons around the globe as a single-step procedure due to its results and benefits, like the low rate of complications, the low maintenance it requires, anatomical conservation of the gastro-esophageal junction as well as the conservation of the exit of the stomach, including the pylorus valve, permitting adequate gastric emptying. Also, the procedure is very attractive due to the lack of mal-absorption and the fact that the intestines are left untouched. Therefore, vitamins and minerals are absorbed in the gastrointestinal track as they normally are.

How does it work?

The gastric sleeve is a stomach resection that works as a restrictive procedure. This means the patient can only intake small amounts of food at a time. The rest of the calories the body needs will come from stored fat in the body. So the result is the patient loses weight. On a scale from 1 to 10,ten being the amount of food a patient currently eats without any weight loss procedure, he or she will be able to eat a3 approximately (depending on the surgeon's technique) with the gastric sleeve. The GS has also a "hormone" factor. The ghrelin is an amino acid, which is secreted in the stomach. The more ghrelin the patient produces the more hunger the patient has. The part of the stomach that is taken out in the gastric sleeve procedure is the part of the stomach that produces the most amount of ghrelin. Therefore, after the surgery is performed, the majority of the patients experience a pronounced decrease in hunger. The decrease in ghrelin has been seen to occur dramatically even after 24 hours of having surgery. Currently, the sleeve is considered by some to be a mixed procedure, not just a restrictive procedure. This means that the patient will only be able to intake very small amounts of food and also has an endocrine (hormonal) element with the reduction of the ghrelin, so the patient feels less hunger.

How is the surgery done?

All the procedures for weight loss that are done through laparoscopy surgery are done with general anesthesia. This permits maximum relaxation of your muscles, giving your surgeon an adequate cavity or space to work in your abdomen resulting in better exposure of the anatomy. When we say "laparoscopy" we talk about minimum invasive surgery that is done through tiny incisions versus traditional surgery which involves a big incision that cut through all the layers in the abdominal wall. Laparoscopy has the benefits of less pain, faster recover, better cosmesis, among other advantages. Once the camera and instruments are inside the abdomen, there is a need for a special instrument to cauterize the vessels that are attached to the greater curvature. There are several instruments for this, but the most popular ones are Ligasure™ from Covidien and the HARMONIC® Scalpel made by Ethicon Endosurgery. These devices carry electrical energy and are transformed into heat that will cauterize the vessels on the instrument preventing bleeding where the surgeon decides to cut. This way the greater curvature of the stomach is mobilized and freed from its attachments. The next step is to introduce a calibration tube or "bougie" that will help serve as a guide to do the stapling/cutting to form the new stomach. This bougie can be of different sizes; the size is expressed in French(Fr) measurement. The larger bougie the surgeon decides to use, the larger the new sleeve will be. The initial sleeves were done as the first surgery of the two-stage operation of a Duodenal Switch. On this initial step, surgeons commonly used large bougies (60 Fr) to create the sleeves. This would give temporary weight loss and a second stage or surgery was needed to complete the Duodenal Switch surgery for adequate weight loss. With time and observation of results, surgeons started using smaller bougies and having better results as a single stage surgery. The most common bougies used today by surgeons are in the range between 32-40 Fr. These bougies have shown to give optimal weight loss and keep the patients in a safe range to avoid any long-term complications like stenosis or strictures.

This bougie is introduced through the patient's mouth during surgery, and the surgeon will orientate the calibration tube toward the smaller curvature. Now that there is a pattern and size to guide the surgeon, the stapling and cutting of the stomach is carried out by a disposable instrument, the stapler, also called Endo-GIA (stands for Gastrointestinal Anasto mosis) and cartridges. There are two main companies that develop this technology. These are Covidien and Ethicon Endosurgery. Both companies carry cartridges that are loaded with three lines of staples on each side and a blade to cut in the middle. Using these loads will permit a staple line to have three micro lines of staples on each side. Then by activating the stapler, the blade will cut in between, keeping a very clean surgical field due to the seal of the stomach that will remain and of the stomach that will be removed. This is carried out numerous times and several cartridges are used to complete the cutting and sealing off of the new stomach from the stomach that will be removed.

After the stapling is complete, some surgeons may or may not suture the staple line depending on personal preference. In our practice, we strongly believe that over sewing the staple line will help prevent any bleeding from the site of the surgery and at the same time give extra support or resistance to the staples themselves. It does consume some time during surgery and some extra laparoscopic sewing techniques to perform this, but with practice this procedure can be performed in 5-10 minutes.

Which is better: Only stapling the stomach or stapling and sewing the stomach?

Once the stapling and cutting of the stomach has been achieved from the starting point (close to the pylorus) to the upper part of the stomach (angle of His) the surgeon has two options.

1. He or she can leave the Gastric Sleeve this way
2. or run a suture over the stapling line.

Studies have shown that the risk of a leak by leaving only the staples may be as high as 6 to 7%. Running the suture over the staple line may decrease the chance of a leak to <1%. Our experience has shown that the risk of a leak over sewing the staple line is <0.32%.

I frequently use the example and explain to my patients that if you were to have a hole in jeans, let's say in the knee area, it is a very different to only place a patch than to place the patch and reinforce by sewing on the edge of it. It will definitely add more resistance to tearing, therefore adding security to the procedure.

Also, when doing the GS procedure the surgeon has the option to staple the stomach using special stapling cartridges. Currently, there are several companies offering the use of buttresses or reinforcement material to each cartridge. This material is usually a very fine and thin layer of bovine tissue or synthetic material that is be placed on each load/cartridge to act as a cushion in between the staples and the stomach wall. The idea of this is to make the staple line more secure, but current trials have not shown any significant results and some authors do criticize the use of the material due to the fact that it will take up some space between the staples and the stomach tissue; therefore, the staples may "grab" less tissue and may not reduce the percentage of leaks.

Testing the sleeve for leaks after it is done is also controversial.

Some surgeons think it's worthless and don't do any type of testing, some do a leak test during surgery involving dyed water. The way this is done is that the sleeve is filled up with methylene blue-dyed water and the staple line is checked for any dyed water. The other test is to fill the sleeve with air and look for bubbles along the staple line. Same principle how a flat tire is checked.

We currently perform both tests (air and dyed water) during surgery to ensure the integrity of the staple line prior to us exiting the abdomen and finishing the procedure. Back in 2006 we started doing leak tests but we would perform these tests the day after surgery. We did over +2500 leak tests and never saw a leak but the thing was that if we would've seen a leak the tendency was take the patient back into the operating room after 24 hours.

Nowadays we check for leaks at that same moment we do the procedure.

It is important to state that even if no leak is present at the time of a leak test it does not mean the patient will be leak-free since there are other factors, like complying with the diet after surgery, excessive inflammation of the sleeve, lower blood supply at the GE junction, etc. that may contribute to a leak after these tests are performed.

Preoperative Diet for the Gastric Sleeve

Before any weight loss surgery, a patient is required to observe a diet based on his/her body mass index (BMI). The patient's weight will determine how long he/she needs to follow the diet. This diet is a preparation phase to ensure that the patient will be in good condition for the surgery. Most patients who are obese have a condition called fatty liver or in medical terms hepatic steatosis. This condition enlarges the liver and makes it heavier. There is a direct relationship between the patient's weight and the liver size. This means that the heavier the patient is, the bigger the liver grows.

If a surgeon were to decide to go into surgery without the patient doing the preoperative diet, there is a chance the surgery would not be possible. Why? Because the liver would be so enlarged and heavy, that it probably wouldn't give the surgeon a chance to visualize the anatomy he has to work on properly. So our goal when we give the patient a preoperative diet is not to starve the patient or make him endure hunger in a bad way; it has the purpose of helping the patient get into a favorable condition for the surgery. This means that if the patient sticks to the diet and goes by the book, he/she will be getting the liver in an optimal condition for the surgery by shrinking it, thus making the surgery possible and having the surgeon manipulate less internally, resulting in a better recovery for the patient.

The preoperative diet that most surgeons give out is based on liquids. This is what the diet prior to the surgery may consist of: strictly liquids. Other surgeons give out a specific diet with shakes that substitute for meals. Others prescribe a diet that is a combination of shakes and liquids.

In our practice, we give out a diet that consists of liquids.

Allowed beverages include some shakes, coffee, tea, sports drinks, and broth; some juices are also permitted, as well as protein supplements.

Our goal is for you to keep your daily calorie intake between 800 and 1000 calories. It usually takes 2-3 days for your hunger to start disappearing. In other words, these 2-3 days are the most difficult part of the diet for some patients. You may have some side effects such as a headache or irritability, especially at the beginning of the diet. This is mainly caused by a reduction in your actual diet to approximately 1,000calories. The average pre-operative patient consumes an average of 4,300 calories per day. Therefore, consuming products with some fiber in them, like the shakes, will also give you some energy and satiety. You can use 100% whey protein powder to make a meal replacement and do that3 times a day and supplement with liquids in between. Mix with skim milk, it tastes better than with water. Constipation may also occur. You just need to make sure you are drinking enough water and try to keep your calorie intake between800-1,000 per day.

The length of the diet is determined by the surgeon and may differ from one patient to another.

In our practice, we determine the length of the diet by the patient's body mass index (BMI) or weight.

- Patients who have a BMI lower than 35 are not required to do a liquid diet prior to surgery because they are less likely to have an enlarged fatty liver.
- Patients who have a BMI from 35 to 42 are

required to do the preoperative diet for 1 week prior to surgery.

- Patients with a BMI between42 and 47 do a 10-day liquid diet
- Patients who have a BMI higher than 47 are required to diet for 14 days prior to surgery.
- Patients who are over 300 lbs are required to diet for3 weeks
- Patients more than 400 lbs for 4 weeks, etc.

These are only some guidelines we use in our practice, but the recommendations from surgeon to surgeon and case to case do vary.

Examples of liquids that are allowed on the pre-op diet:

- Black Coffee
- Tea/iced tea
- Low or no sugar fruit juices
- Jell-O®-sugar free
- Water
- Gatorade®
- Sports Drinks
- Crystal Light®
- Slim-Fast® Low Carb Shakes
- Atkins™ Advantage Shakes
- Beef, vegetable, or chicken broth
- Propel® Flavored Water
- Any 100% whey protein powder mixed with water or skim milk
- Popsicles®-sugar free
- Sugar-Free Kool-Aid®,Tang® etc.
- Carnation® Instant Breakfast-sugar free made

Chapter 4

The Surgery

*(The following information may vary
from surgical practice to surgical practice.)*

At our center, the average time to complete a gastric sleeve surgery is approximately 25-35 minutes.

This average time was not like this at the beginning when I began performing this procedure and my average time to complete a sleeve was an hour to an hour and 20 minutes.

I have been blessed to work with the same surgical team, including anesthesiologists, doctors, OR nurses, assistants, etc. on every single case, every single day for many years now. This means that everyone knows their part - what to do, when to do it - avoiding any lost time in preparing, setting up, explaining steps to follow, etc. I like to see it as a musical orchestra that plays the same melody every day, year after year. Everyone know it by heart!

As we continued to focus on the gastric sleeve and perfected our technique, we were able to lower the operating time with great benefit for our patients.

The less time in the operating room the better outcomes for patients and less risk of complications too.

We don't routinely use drains or urinary catheters in our patients since the procedure is so short (anybody can last 35 minutes without the need to pee) and we double test for leaks prior to finishing the procedure.

Sometimes people ask me about the use of drains. Why don't I use them routinely?

Well, back when I started performing the procedure I routinely used drains in my first 250 patients but not anymore. Since the sleeve is (should be) a very clean procedure, there is nothing to drain once the procedure is done since the stomach is sealed. The use of a drains may be an entrance point for bacteria to the abdominal cavity or in some cases maybe misleading.

Let me explain a bit more on this.

Sometimes surgeons leave a drain with the intention to detect a leak at an early point, but regular drains left after the gastric sleeve procedure do not "drain" a leak adequately.

Why?

When a leak is present, a thick slime is what usually builds up inside the abdomen and this thick consistency of the fluid will clog the drain.

Surgeons may think that everything is "OK" since nothing is coming out from the drain but a leak maybe present. So what we do is check for leaks prior to finishing the sleeve surgery and after that we constantly check patients through the following days looking out for clinical signs and symptoms that are more reliable than a drain.

Remember, a leak usually happens the following days after surgery, so *it's also up to you to play your role in take care of your new stomach by following your doctor's guidelines.*

On your surgery day and after you are admitted to the hospital, you will be taken into the operating room. To avoid stress, tension and or anxiety, we routinely pre-medicate patients once they are evaluated by the anesthesiologist. This means patients are given medication in their IV to help them relax and take the edge off.

Most patients may not even remember when they are taken to the operating room and may only remember once they are in the recovery room or back in their rooms. This makes is so easy for patients and it's practically stress-free.

The first 24 hours.

Right after surgery you will continue to receive medications and fluids through your IV line to keep you in great shape. Sometimes you may experience a dry mouth sensation that is a side-effect of a medication (atropine) used with the anesthesia that will dry your mouth and throat, this will actually help your anesthesiologist deal with less saliva and you will have a much clearer airway during and after surgery. This effect may continue the following hours after surgery and some patients wake up with a dry mouth.

At this point it is recommend that rinse your mouth, you may brush your teeth if you prefer, but don't swallow any water until your surgeon indicates so.

In our practice, I like for my patients to let the stomach rest until the following morning and we maintain good hydration through the IV.

The first 24 hours following the procedure I routinely schedule medications for my patients that include medication for pain, nausea, inflammation, heartburn, antibiotics, blood thinners, etc. This keeps patients in the best shape possible. At this point patients are moving out of bed by themselves, getting up to the bathroom and doing some walking on the halls that same day.

Day after surgery.

The following morning we place a heparin lock where the IV is, patients are walking the halls and they are able to take a shower too if preferred. The heparin lock gives the patients a lot of freedom to move around but at the same time keeps the vein accessible in case we need medication for the following hours. Usually at this point patients go with medications as needed and if all is well we remove the IV completely later that day. I tell patients that this day is dedicated to 5 things:

1.- sucking on ice
2.- walking
3.- resting
4.- the sleeve blush
5.- going home

Sucking on ice.

The idea of having ice the following day after surgery is real simple. The cold of the ice is excellent for inflammation or swollen tissue. Remember when you were a kid and you would bump a knee or your forehead? The most common thing was that your mom would place an ice pack on it to help the swollen tissue come down fast. The same idea follows after gastric sleeve surgery. Inflammation of the stomach is important since the stomach was manipulated, stapled, etc. So the ice comes into play and is very important following surgery. The idea is for you to put a piece of ice in your mouth and let it melt. Only swallow whatever is melting and avoid taking chunks of ice. This way the melting ice will become cold water which is what will eventually help the sleeve get in better shape right after surgery plus helping with the hydration too.

Walking

Walking after surgery is important. Take advantage of having your surgery through laparoscopy (minimal invasive surgery). This gives you a fast recovery. Most patients are able to get up by themselves that same day after surgery to the bathroom and walking the halls that same afternoon or evening.

- Walking helps by promoting venous return of blood in your legs, reducing the chance of deep vein thrombosis, etc.
- Walking also promotes your intestines to move a

better pace helping you reduce nausea and bloating of your abdomen.

- Walking is encourage the following day after surgery and normally patients walk the halls 2 or 3 times every 30-60 minutes.
- Throughout the day patients can take naps and rest followed by more walking. As you can see walking is an important thing after surgery to be sure to put some effort here.

Resting

The first night following surgery patients usually don't get much sleep. Normally patients after surgery sleep or rest for the following hours and sometimes this causes patients to be up easily over the night. We know about this, therefore patients are allowed to nap throughout the following day to make up for some sleep to help them catch up to their own sleeping cycle.

The sleeve blush.

There is something I always explain to patients the following day after surgery and we call it the "sleeve blush". That same afternoon you have surgery or the following day you may develop a red/warm face, neck and even part or your arms. This is expected especially on very white-skin people. It's important to state that not everybody develops this sleeve blush. Darker-skin people may fell the warm the sleeve blush in the same areas. Patients should be aware that the sleeve blush is just temporary and lasts between 24 and 48 hours. It has a direct relationship with the swollen tissue of the sleeve. As the swollen tissue starts to come down the blush disappears. Please note that feeling your face warm does not indicate you have a fever or a reaction to a medication, as most patients would think. The sleeve blush produces this but will not elevate your complete body's temperature as when you have fever.

Going home

Depending on your surgeon's practice you will be going home probably after 24-48 hours after your surgery. We normally discharge or local/regional patients after 24 hours but our out-of-town patients are discharged from our care after 48 hours. This gives us an extra 24 hours of surveillance of any issue that may arise the first couple of days after surgery. On discharge our out-of-town patients will be staying an extra night at a hotel or catching a plane back home. It is important to mention that from this point forward the most important thing on behalf of the patient is to stick to the guidelines and diet phases 100%. The integrity of the sleeve depends on this and following the rules is crucial. Keep in mind that after your sleeve has healed you will enjoy the benefits of your procedure and weight loss but in the meant time the following diet phases will help your sleeve healed correctly. The following pages will help you understand these phases and what is to follow after your sleeve.

Chapter 5

Postoperative Weight Loss Guide for Gastric Sleeve Patients

This chapter will help guide you through the weeks and months ahead. These are the basic tools to help you be as successful as you can be. The rest is up to you. *Compliance is the key to your success and well-being.*

Important tips to remember for successful weight loss

The greatest weight loss will occur within the first six to nine months. It will start to slow after that, but can continue for a total of 12-18 months or more. You may intermittently have plateaus or stalls in your weight loss that may last up to a month. This is usually an indication that you are eating too many carbohydrates or calories and/or not exercising enough. Take this as a sign to re-examine your eating and exercise habits. Most patients' weight will plateau after 8-12 months. After this time, additional weight loss may be difficult, so take advantage of what I call the "golden year," which is the first 12 months. Weight regain may also occur if too many calories are consumed, exercise is discontinued or old habits, such as grazing, snacking, or poor eating habits return.

Consumption of fluids

- Consumption of an adequate amount of liquid, preferably water, is crucial.

- Patients should consume a minimum of 2 - 2½ quarts (64-80 fluid ounces) of liquids per day. This should be done slowly and throughout the day. The easiest way to keep track of this is to purchase a 32-ounce water bottle. Use the sports cap on top for easier consumption and less air intake, and finish at least 2 bottles of liquids a day. Sip, sip, sip . . . It may take a couple of weeks to build up to this amount; the main thing is to continually have that something in your hand to drink.

- This amount should be increased by 10-20% when the weather is very hot and humid to prevent dehydration.

- The first 2 or 3 days after surgery it may be difficult to get enough water in unless you use a trick. You need to take a tiny sip of water and wait 2-3 minutes. Then sip again. You should do this while you are away from home during the day. By doing this, you'll be able to get enough water. If you don't do this and you wait until you're thirsty, you will fall behind on your liquids and you will not be able to gulp water down at this point. So remember the sip-wait technique!

- During the initial week it is important to look at the color of your urine. If it starts to look darker than usual you are falling behind on liquids and you will need to push a little harder to consume at least 64 ounces.

- In the first 30-45 days after surgery, avoid drinking more than 3-4 ounces of liquids (⅓ of a cup) in a 10-minute period to avoid vomiting or uncomfortable sensations. <u>Avoid gulping</u> any more than1 ounce (shot glass size) <u>at a time.</u> Eventually, you may be able to drink more at a time.

Solid foods

It is VERY important that as a patient you must understand the following: You <u>should</u> <u>not</u> <u>eat</u> absolutely <u>anything solid for the following 21 days following your surgery</u>. These are my guidelines and you should follow your doctor's guidelines. In our practice we take care of your well-crafted sleeve and we want you to keep the way we left it in the operating room. You must follow the liquid phases after your surgery so that the sleeve heals in a correct manner. Believe me it is worth it! If you do not comply with this you are placing yourself at risk with possible damage to your sleeve, causing irritation, swollen tissue or even a leak. Here is where I want you to understand that it is worth waiting: If you develop a leak you will be an NPO (nothing by mouth) for weeks, you'll be back in the hospital, taken back in the operating room or intensive care unit probably fed the following weeks either by a feeding tube or your vein (total parenteral nutrition line). I'm not trying to give you the worst scenario here but I do want you to understand that we have a reason for you to follow guidelines. As I tell my patients, nobody will be watching you 24/7 like baby so whatever you put in your mouth make sure it is permitted.

No solid food the following 3 weeks after surgery. Your stomach is healing.

- Once solids are permitted, they are usually consumed 3 times per day. (This should correspond to mealtimes.) Some patients will need to eat 5-6 times per day in small amounts in order to get in adequate protein and calories, so 3 times per day is merely a guideline, you should adjust your needs accordingly.
- Snacking between meals or "grazing" on small amounts of food throughout the day may sabotage your attempts at successful weight loss.
- If you "graze," you will not lose an adequate amount of weight because you may consume too many calories.
- You will need to be the judge of your meals and snacks. Some patients need to have 5 mini-

meals per day and that works for them. Since everyone is an individual, there is no hard and fast rule. You have to do what works best for you.

Protein for nutrition

- As with any weight loss procedure, the primary source of nutrition should be protein.
- 70%-75% of all calories consumed should be protein based(eggs, fish, lean meats, etc.; bacon is not a lean meat).
- Carbohydrates (bread, rice, pasta, potatoes, beans, sugar etc.) should make up only about 10%-20%, and fats (butter, cheese, etc.) only 5%-15% of the calories that you eat. If you must eat the carbs, opt for quality whole grains. Use this guideline only to start off the solid phase but as you progress and get the hang of the following months I would advise to focus on your protein THEN fat and keep your carb intake under 30 gr per day.
- A diet consisting of 600-800 calories and about 60-70 grams of protein should be your goal for at least the first6months. Caloric intake can

increase as your stomach stretches a bit (which is normal and expected).

- Swollen ankles, fatigue, hair loss, cracked nails, and defective healing and immunity are just some of the side effects of inadequate protein consumption (not to mention difficulty losing weight). Hair loss may also be due to hormonal changes, but protein levels can be checked to be sure you are not developing a protein deficiency.

Avoid combining liquids and solid foods

- NEVER drink liquids when eating solid foods (at least the first 6-8 months after surgery). Even though this will not harm your sleeve if you decide to drink and eat at the same time, it does produce a very uncomfortable sensation in patients that I would like for you to avoid.

- Liquids should be avoided for a period of 15-30 minutes before and 30-45 minutes after eating solid food or meals. The reason for this is that the sleeve acts as a funnel and if you eat the food will start to pack itself in the new sleeve. If at this point you drink some liquids, by gravity, it will try to work itself down to the bottom of the sleeve interchanging or moving the solid food. This may cause this sensation I'm trying for you to avoid that can be described as chest pressure, food stuck with no progress forward nor backward, abdominal pain among other symptoms. After 6-8 months you may give it a try and some patients are able to tolerate it fairly well. Prior to those 6-8 months, don't give it a try!

Use of sugar

I'm not a fan of sugar at all! In fact you'll notice that I push my patients to transform themselves to a low carb freak once they dominate the low calorie diet the following weeks/months after the surgery. In other words you can use sugar/carbs initially the first few weeks after surgery. This avoids headaches, dizziness, low energy, etc. Once your body accommodates the low-calorie input you can then start moving away from carbohydrates and make protein and fat your new best friends. This will assure you the most amazing weight loss possible by having just a few calories per day (the sleeve's job) and you'll be forcing your body to burn stored fat and turning it into carbs (by lowering your carb intake to under 30 gr per day). Please, please avoid foods that contain sugar, especially simple sugars such as those found in most sodas, fruit juices, desserts, candy, etc. Also avoid carbohydrates such as bread, crackers, rice, pasta, and potatoes. Avoid the "orange vegetables" like carrots and sweet potatoes, as they are high in sugar. If you must eat the carbs, opt for whole grains and 100% whole wheat products, brown rice, etc.

Believe me it will make a huge difference down the road. Without even knowing, avoiding sugar will become a habit, all you have to do is focus.

Overall focus for foods

- You must focus on eating enough protein to prevent malnutrition and hair loss. If you eat protein rich foods first at each meal, you will have little room left in your stomach for simple sugars. Also eating a good amount of protein will protect your muscles too while you are losing weight and that way it will come off mainly from your stored fat.

Things you must remember:

- Sugar and other carbohydrates may slow your weight loss because they are so easily digested and absorbed. Gastric sleeve patients who have early plateaus are most always consuming too many carbohydrates. Because the negative biofeedback of dumping syndrome is normally not present with this operation, it is all too easy to start eating too much sugar and other carbohydrates. Eating protein first and when hungry will help to minimize the chance of consuming too many carbohydrates. Believe me down the road you'll feel better too!

- Sugar, sugar alcohols, and artificial sweeteners cause gas, bloating, and diarrhea. Gastric sleeve patients usually do not develop dumping issues; however, they may if they eat significant amounts of fat or sugar. If too much sugar is consumed, it may enter the intestines rapidly and travel through quickly. This may lead to gas, bloating, and a mad dash for the bathroom. This is also seen in some patients with very rich liquids, especially with thick liquids or shakes during the initial phases.

- Avoid starchy foods such as rice, pasta, cereals, and mashed potatoes. Again, these are carbohydrates and will slow your weight loss.

Learn to recognize feeling full

Stop eating/drinking when you begin to feel full. Do not "stuff" yourself. This may cause your stomach pouch to stretch. Learn to recognize that signal of beginning fullness.

Begin an exercise program

You should begin an exercise program. You will accelerate your weight loss and have a better chance of reaching your goal weight by establishing a good aerobic exercise program and making healthy dietary choices. In addition, and more importantly, aerobic exercise strengthens the heart and makes you feel better. It can also help to suppress hunger. We'll talk more about exercise later in this book.

Weight plateaus

As mentioned above, patients whose weight loss has hit a plateau are usually eating too many carbohydrates.

Lack of exercise may also limit the amount of weight loss. Occasionally, patients who exercise a great deal can experience a weight plateau due to increased muscle and lean body mass (like body-builders). Remember—muscle is denser than fat and thus weighs more. These patients often notice that they are losing inches and clothing sizes and should keep up the good work! Weight loss through exercise is the healthiest way to lose! Ask yourself if you are losing inches or if your clothes are feeling loose.

Avoid the scale

- STAY OFF THE SCALE! Use your clothes and how they fit as a guide. If you must weigh, try to pick 1 day of the week and stick to it. Otherwise, it may drive you crazy and you will only sabotage yourself and your thinking.

- Take a monthly photo; this is a better indicator than the scale. Also, it is important that you remind yourself that this is your own journey and you shouldn't compare yourself to others who've had the same or another weight loss procedure.

- Do not let the scale dictate your progress for you.

Tips for eating

- Remember that the most difficult (and most important) time after surgery is the first 3-6 months. This is also the most important time because the habits that you develop in this period will be the ones that you will probably adopt for the rest of your life. In the first months after surgery, you are relearning how much you can eat (portion size as well as "bite" size), how well you have to chew, and what you can eat without developing problems. Although everyone is different, usually by the sixth month patients are eating most regular (healthy) foods—but in much smaller portions than they did before surgery. There will definitely be foods that you will never want to eat again because they will cause some type of "intestinal distress." As a reminder, the following tips should be useful:

✻ Always eat protein or protein rich foods first during your meals. Good sources of protein include fish, shrimp, eggs, soy, skim milk, and lean meats. Potatoes, rice, and cereals are NOT good sources of protein. A very good rule of thumb also is to always remember "Eat Protein & Produce." If you can remember these two things, you will be very successful.

- It is recommended that you DO NOT drink carbonated beverages. If you must, let them go flat before consuming.

11 basic Guidelines For Success

1. I will exercise 5 times per week for 30-45 minutes.
2. I will watch my intake of carbohydrates.
3. I will try to eat 3-5 small meals per day & no unhealthy snacks between meals.
4. I will drink at least 8 glasses of water each day. (This will be difficult the first few months)
5. I will eat a minimum of 60-70 grams of protein each day.
6. I will honor my commitment to good health and healthy choices.
7. I will have follow-up appointments with my

doctor as needed.

8. I will always take my vitamins and supplements.
9. I will weigh myself no more than once-a-week.
10. I will remember that this is my own journey and not compare myself to others. Remember everybody is different.
11. I will always keep in my mind that practicing my new habits will make me healthier, happier, stronger and more energetic.

Vitamins and supplements

By having undergone the gastric sleeve procedure, you have committed yourself to a lifetime of making sure you eat right. Oftentimes we don't take in enough vitamins and minerals. Therefore, it is recommended that you take a multivitamin daily. Please check with your surgeon for his/her recommendations and doses.

Multivitamins

* Multivitamins (with folate and iron): we recommend one or two adult doses daily.
* Comprehensive Multivitamins (chewable, liquid, or gummy if you choose)
* You may also try Centrum® Performance tablets

or liquid form, Flintstones®, Costco® vitamins, One A Day* gummies, etc. All these are over-the- counter and do not require a prescription. You can certainly purchase the equivalent to name brand products in most drugstores.

- Menstruating women or patients with anemia should take a multivitamin with supplemental iron.

- ✱ Your multivitamin must contain folate or folic acid. A dose of 400 mcg a day is essential! It will be listed on the label.

Vitamin B12

- Vitamin B12 deficiency can cause anemia as well as serious neurological problems.

- B12 deficiency is rare but has sometimes been reported with a restrictive surgery such as the gastric sleeve. We do recommend supplemental B12. This may be taken in your choice of forms: sublingual (under your tongue), intramuscular, or the recently-developed intranasal administration.

Calcium

✳ Calcium/vitamin D complex is important, especially in women, to prevent osteoporosis and we recommend it as a supplement for the gastric sleeve procedure.

General guidelines: Liquids and solids

Liquids

- Only clear liquids should be consumed for at least the first 7 days after surgery (starting on your discharge day from the hospital). These are liquids that can easily pass through a straw. These should always go down easily and be tolerated without problems. If you can't tolerate liquids and are vomiting them, your surgeon needs to know. Contact him or her immediately. Some patients have pain when drinking cold water, so try warm or room temperature water or decaffeinated green tea. We are aware that many surgeons let their patients advance to solid foods more rapidly. We are strongly opposed to this because solid foods in the first three weeks may lead to forceful vomiting or retching. This vomiting can cause a disruption in the sutures or staples and lead to an emergency reoperation, long hospital stay, and possibly even death.

Here are some personal recommendations:

- **Avoid carbonated beverages** because they can expand your stomach with the gas and cause abdominal distension and even severe pain.

- **Avoid caffeinated beverages** until you are at least 2-3 weeks post-op—they can cause dehydration. A good rule of thumb is as follows: If you are consistently able to drink 2 quarts of liquid each day, it is OK to drink de-caffeinated beverages as soon as 10 days post-op, which includes decaf coffee or teas. Drinking coffee too soon may cause nausea or vomiting or even swelling of the sleeve.

- **Drink lots of water** using a sport bottle to avoid swallowing air. Early on, you will probably need to drink small amounts frequently since your stomach will not accept larger amounts. There is no magic number, but 8 glasses of water per day should suffice. If the weather is hot and/or humid, you may require 1 or 2 more glasses each day. You can drink a shot glass of water or protein drink every 5-10 minutes as a way to control the volume you put into your stomach. You will notice if you are dehydrated because your mouth will be dry, your lips will be dry, and your urine will be dark and of less volume. These should be reminders to drink more and that you are falling behind on fluid intake.

- **Sugar-free drinks are best.** Never think that any "juice" drink is healthy. If it is a juice drink, it most likely is loaded with sugar. For example, apple juice is very high in sugar. "Natural" juice contains natural sugar, and many juice drinks contain additional added sugars. Sugar free Tang, Crystal Light, and Diet Snapple are popular with many of our patients and are fine to drink after surgery.

- **Sugar-free Popsicles® and sugar-free Jell-O®** are fine to consume. They help break-up the monotony of this diet phase.

- **Do not consume liquids and solids at the same time.** If you do, you could vomit. Sip fluids slowly 30-45 minutes after a meal. Stop drinking liquids 15-30 minutes before the next meal.

- **Green tea** (decaffeinated) works well for nausea, especially warm teas.

- **Milk:** Some adults cannot digest lactose in milk, and some obesity surgery patients become intolerant of milk after surgery. Your small intestine needs the enzyme lactase to break down the lactose in milk so it can be absorbed. If you do not have enough enzymes for the amount of milk consumed, you may not be able to break down all the lactose, and this could lead to bloating, flatulence (gas), crampy abdominal pain, and even diarrhea. You will probably be able to tolerate up to a cup of milk after surgery, but be cautious and watch for side effects. Try lactose-free milk or lactase tablets, such as Lactaid® or Dairy Ease®. Milk and dairy products should always be skim or fat-free.

- **Remember:** you should try to consume 60-70 grams of protein each day. In the liquid dietary phase, you may supplement with your protein drinks.

Solids

Work up to these gradually. Solid food should not be eaten for the first 3 weeks following surgery. Soft foods, such as eggs, tofu, yogurt, etc., may be introduced at the 3-week point, and should go down easily before solid food is attempted. Be cautious and don't eat too much or too fast. Your suture and staple line is usually healed at the 10-14 post-op day. That is why it is so important to make sure things are soft and go down easily, since you may disrupt your staple lines. We have seen this in patients who chose to eat regular food in the first 1-2 weeks after surgery, so please follow your surgeon's dietary instructions carefully. Bite size should be half of what you are used to; use a toddler spoon if you need to for visualization purposes, and you should chew the food twice as long until it is well pulverized.

Remember: Digestion begins in your mouth by chewing very well.

In the first month on solid foods, you should feel satisfied or full with a very small portion of food (e.g., one to two ounces of tuna, or one egg). Meals like this should take 30 minutes to consume. Eating any faster may cause vomiting. If you are having difficulty or have a significant amount of dietary intolerance, please contact your doctor's office.

Here are some personal recommendations:

- **Always set out small size meals.** Use your measuring cups . . .do not start with a large meal and think that you will just eat a smaller amount. You will always eat more than you should. Place food on a small plate or saucer and use small utensils such as baby spoons or a seafood fork. Your eyes are still bigger than your stomach, so don't "eat" with your eyes. □

- **Portion tips:**
  - 3 ounces = the size of a deck of cards or a woman's palm.
  - ¼ cup = one layer on your hand or the size of a golf ball
  - 2 tablespoons = the size of a golf ball
  - 1 ounce = the size of 4 dice or a 1 inch ice cube
  - ½ cup = the size of a small wallet or compact case

- **While some fruits are okay to eat** (bananas, strawberries, raspberries, blueberries, watermelon, and blackberries), please avoid fruit juices or processed fruit products as they are high in sugar content.

- **Eggs are okay** in just about any form.
- **Baked fish products,** especially fish fillets, are quick and easy to make and a good source of protein.
- **Peanut butter and peanuts** are high in calories and they should be avoided. Soy nuts are a much better choice. A few almonds are a good source of protein and good fat too.
- **Tofu** is a good source of protein.
- **You may want to use a blender** for anything that seems too solid to go down easily and stay down.
- **Most soups are okay,** but they may need to be pureed. Cream soups are higher in fat and should be avoided unless the label specifies "fat-free." Do not eat soups with noodles or rice; stick to the meat and veggie varieties.
- **Pork tenderloin, steak, turkey, ostrich, and chicken** are all good sources of protein.
- **Canned fish products** (tuna, crab, salmon) are a good protein source. You may wish to

prepare them in low-fat ways with olive oil or mustard. Avoid mayonnaise unless it is low fat or fat-free.

- **Turkey and beef jerky** are good sources of protein and may serve as good protein-rich snacks. Make sure to chew well.

- **Lean deli meats** (sliced thinly) are high in protein and are well tolerated by most patients.

- **Protein bars and drinks.** The protein sources for these include everything from whey protein and milk-protein isolate to soy protein. These bars are dense, and they may cause gas, bloating, and diarrhea. If you have trouble with a particular bar, try one with another type of protein. Pure Protein® Bars are excellent bars that taste good. GNC and other health food stores have many different kinds. Be sure to read the labels and choose low-carb, low sugar products.

✳ **Remember these two words, Protein & Produce**—your two new best friends.

Chapter 6

Postoperative Phases of Diet Progression

(Note: These phases may vary depending on your surgeon and his or her guidelines.)

The size of your stomach has been reduced from about 60 ounces to 3-4 ounces.

In order to prevent discomfort and stretching, and to protect the integrity of the pouch, you should follow these recommendations as closely as possible.

The dietary plan following a gastric sleeve procedure is broken down into four phases:

1. Clear Liquids (Phase 1),
2. Full Liquids (Phase 2),
3. Soft Foods (Phase 3), and
4. Solid or Regular Foods (Phase 4).

You must remain on clear liquids for at least 7 days after surgery; this starts on your discharge day from the hospital. Diet progression after three weeks varies from patient to patient. These precautions minimize the chance of severe vomiting and disruption of staples or stitches. After 3 weeks, healing is complete enough to progress to soft foods.

NOTE: You may progress to the next phase only after waiting the minimum amount of time and after feeling completely comfortable with the previous phase (no vomiting or nausea). If, after advancing to the next phase, you develop problems, go back to liquids and advance only after you have tolerated liquids without any problems for 48 hours.

Phase 1: Liquids (first 7 days) - NO SOLID FOOD!

During your first week post-surgery, your diet will consist of thin/clear liquids. The clear liquid diet helps to keep you hydrated and helps to get the body ready to use food after surgery. Your goal this first week is to remember to get in 64 oz. of fluids per day. Let me remind you that the first few days after surgery it will be nearly impossible to do so since your stomach is so swollen. Sip, wait, sip wait! Remember: Any Sugar-free Jell-O®, Sugar-free Popsicles®, and Sugar-free Crystal Light® also count towards your liquid fluid intake. You should sip all day long with this phase to get your required fluids. *If you lack some energy or feel weak or dizzy you may take during this phase liquids that have carbs or sugar in them since they are a good source of calories and you'll need them at this point. Down the road, once you start eating, carbs/sugar will be your enemy.*

- **Thin/clear liquids** are items that you can easily drink through a straw: Some suggestions are noted below.
    - Water
    - 100% Whey Protein Isolite Bullets® 42 or 25 gram
    - Propel Water®
    - Ice chips
    - Flavored water
    - Chicken or beef broth
    - Consommé
    - Skim milk

- Sugar-free or regular Jell-O®
- Sugar-free or regular Popsicles®
- Crystal Light®, Sugar-free or regular powdered drinks like Tang®
- Mild tea (no cinnamon), green teas
- Low-sugar apple juice, cranberry juice
- Fruit ices (without chunks of fruit)
- Sugar-free Kool-Aid®

- **Avoid caffeine or carbonated beverages.** These will cause unpleasant side effects and may also cause complications.

- **Drink a minimum of 2 quarts of liquids** throughout the day to prevent dehydration.

- **Sip at your own pace.** Don't think that if your stomach is now a 4 oz stomach it will only hold 4 oz. Remember that your stomach has an exit and fluid is able to flow through your stomach with ease. You set the pace.

- **Always sip**—never gulp or drink quickly. Gulping or drinking more fluids in a short period of time will be possible a few weeks down the road once the swelling of the sleeve goes away.

- **Keep track of your daily intake** to be

certain you get enough liquids and protein. If it's hot or humid outside and you are sweating, you will need to increase this amount by 10-20%.

- **If your urine is dark or your mouth is dry** or if you feel dizzy, you are not drinking enough. Focus on your fluid intake!

Phase 2: Full liquids (weeks 2 & 3) NO SOLID FOOD!

The full liquid diet is a temporary transition phase between clear liquids and the soft food diet. It is a diet to keep your body hydrated and to help get your body ready for food after surgery. Consume a small amount at first and see how your stomach handles it. You can continue to sip fluids all day with this phase as well. It is important to note whether your protein drink is soy or whey protein based. Some patients may not tolerate one and may want to switch to the other. Remember your goal is to take in 60-70 grams of protein and 64 oz. of fluids per day. In drinking the protein drinks, you are well on your way to fulfilling both goals. You may also continue to have all the items under the clear liquid diet as well.

- **You must stay in this phase for 2 weeks.**
- **If you are lactose intolerant, you may use soy, almond or rice milk instead of cow's milk.**
- Some ideas for the full liquid stage:
  - Milk - skim, 1% or 2 %
  - Soy beverages
  - Fruit juices without the pulp (low-sugar versions)
  - Plain sugar free gelatin

Creamed soups - blended so no chunks are present(these tend to be higher in calories, so watch the content; use low-fat or fat-free versions)

NOTE: Avoid tomato soup for the first couple of weeks due to acid production.

- **TIPS for this phase (full liquids):**
  - Chunky soups - put in the blender and thin out with liquid (broth or water) (Use the meat and veggie types, not pastas or rice varieties.)
- Drinkable yogurt without fruit chunks
- Blended fruit smoothies

- Carnation® Instant Breakfast
- Ice milk
- Popsicles® made from sugar-free juices
- Egg custard - thin
    - Whey protein shakes or any protein shake that gives you 15-20 grams of protein per serving.
- V-8® Juice
- Sugar-free hot cocoa
- Aktins® Advantage Shakes
- Slim-Fast® Low-Carb Shakes
- 100% whey protein powder
- Applesauce
- Labrada® RTD Protein Shakes
- Hood® Low-Carb Chocolate Milk beverage -use with your protein powder to make a great shake(Walmart® carries these in the dairy section)
- **Drink a high quality, liquid protein supplement** of your choice, e.g., Body Fortress® 100% Whey Protein Powder,100% any whey protein powder, Isopure ®, Nectar® or Unjury® products in order to achieve 60-70 grams of protein each day. You may continue to

use the 100% Whey Protein Isolite Bullets®, which will give you 25 or 42 grams of Isolized protein in about 3 oz. tubes. Look for supplements that have more than 15 grams of protein, less than 5 grams of carbohydrates per serving and fewer than 130 calories. Men should probably consume more protein than women— 75-80 grams of protein per day. Be aware that this is sometimes very difficult in the first month but will become easier after that. There are many products out on the market, some good tasting and others not so much. See if you can try samples of products before purchasing a large container you may never finish.

Phase 3: Soft food diet(week 4 after 3 weeks of clear & full liquids) You will do this phase for 1 week

The soft diet serves as a transition from liquids to a regular diet. You can still have all the things on the clear liquid and full liquid diet too.

- **Some suggested soft foods might include the following:**
  - Scrambled eggs (soft, boiled, poached)
  - Egg salad
  - Tuna fish moistened well with low-fat mayo
  - Chicken salad, salmon moistened with low-fat mayo(no celery or hard pieces of veggie)
  - Cottage cheese
  - Mild low-fat cheese
  - Mashed, canned, or cooked fruit
  - Mashed, canned, or well-cooked veggies
  - Refried beans with a bit of low-fat cheese
  - Meats pressure cooked to tenderize
  - Soft fresh banana
  - An occasional mashed sweet potato
  - Yogurt
  - Occasional baked, mashed potatoes (yes, these are carbs, but your body does need some)

- **We recommend 3 meals per day.** However, there may be times when you need a snack in between meals, especially if you are very active. This snack should be a low calorie one, preferably protein food. Examples of healthy snacks include these: a low fat cheese stick, yogurt, soft boiled egg, etc. Do not eat anything solid, blended, or soft again until your next meal time.

- **Eat until you begin to feel full and then stop!** Do not force yourself to finish the food on your plate. Eat until you are comfortable. Do not "stuff" foods down. This may cause your stomach to become overfilled and may be very uncomfortable. You may not lose as much weight in the long run. Never place more food on your plate than you are permitted to eat.

  Measure out half-cup portions of your foods to get an idea of how much you are consuming. It will take time to learn to be able to eyeball food amounts.

- **NEVER start eating solid foods sooner than 1 month after surgery.**

Always remember that with any new food that you try, eat a small amount at first and see how your stomach handles it. Proceed to eat slowly throughout your entire meal. You are aiming for the following:

- **LOW CARB**
- **LOW FAT**
- **LOW SUGAR**
- **HIGH PROTEIN!**

1. You should always stick to the rules regarding the composition of your food, as stated earlier: 60-70 grams of protein and minimal amounts of carbohydrates and fat.

2. Try to read labels and make it a habit to determine how many calories each food contains and how those calories are broken down (percentage from fats, carbohydrates, and protein).

3. Remember that you should eat three meals per day. You shouldn't "graze." Some patients feel better eating 5 very small meals per day, which is fine too since everyone is different and there is no hard and fast rule. Just remember that everything you eat contributes to your overall calorie count for the day. Anytime you eat something blended, soft, or solid it should count as one of your meals. Once you feel yourself getting full, you should stop eating and not resume consuming anything other than a liquid until the next mealtime.

4. Choose soft-textured and moist foods that are easy to chew. For example, eggs (soft boiled or scrambled), tofu, light/no fat yogurt (no chunks of fruit/seeds), and small curd cottage cheese, egg custard.

5. Add non-fat powdered milk or unflavored protein powder to foods (eggs, soups, and yogurt) for extra protein.

6. Never eat more than 4 ounces (½ cup) at one time. Take very small bites and eat slowly. Chew carefully until mushy. You should not eat any foods that are hard to chew or swallow. You may wish to blend foods that are too hard to eat.

7. Remember not to eat and drink at the same time.

8. Between meals, you may drink any thin liquid or liquid protein supplement that you like, provided it doesn't contain sugar, carbonation or fat.

9. Continue to eat between 600-800 calories per day. Weigh yourself weekly to be sure you do not regain or lose too much weight.

10. Introduce one new food each day. Some foods may not go down well and regurgitation may occur. By selecting one new food each day, you will be able to identify which food may have caused problems. The most common food intolerances are red meat, chicken, and bread; meats are better tolerated if moistened with broth.

If you are regularly having problems with vomiting or regurgitation, contact your doctor's office.

Things to remember:

1. The best protein sources to eat are fish, skinless/boneless poultry, eggs, and tofu. These have high protein and low carbohydrate and fat content.

2. Increase the variety of foods you are eating.

Start with one teaspoon of a new food every two days. Beef may not be tolerated well for several months.

3. You should never try to eat more than 4 ounces (volume) at a time. Measure your food (two tablespoons is equal to one ounce, 4 oz = ½ cup). Use small plates as a visual cue to assist you with portion control. Avoid rice, pasta, potatoes, bread, and popcorn. Continue to focus on consuming protein, and stay away from carbohydrates and fats.

4. Avoid food that is high in carbohydrates. After you start eating and have tried different types of food you should start to watch out for the carbs in food. This is very important and will assure you a sustained weight loss. Make it a habit!

5. You should continue to drink 2 quarts of liquids per day, but only between meals. Again, eat 600-800 total calories per day.

6. Avoid eating within 3 hours of going to bed.

7. Choose flavorful foods, since there is no need for picking just bland foods. Experiment with spices lightly at first.

8. Be cautious with seeds, skins, or spicy foods; these may be harder to digest.

9. Your daily intake of carbohydrates should still be less than30 grams. This is the key!

Phase 4: Regular solid food (beginning week 5)

Starting to eat regular solid food like you used to do prior to surgery comes a few weeks after surgery. The importance of starting with a liquid diet and progressing to this phase is crucial to keeping the gastric sleeve in "good shape" while it heals. Following these phases or progression of the diet will avoid tension and stress on the staple line, letting it heal in a better way and lowering the possibility of a major complication like a leak during this period. Getting to week 5 involves eating the way you are going to eat the rest of your life. You need to eat slowly, "listen" to your sleeve and how it handles certain types of food. It is a learning curve that everyone has to go through, and you will learn to live with healthier eating habits that will make a huge change in your life and bring amazing results.

One year after surgery

Here are some pointers you should remember to keep you and your sleeve in a good shape.

- **You should be eating three to five small meals a day.**
- **You should not eat more than 4-6 ounces per meal.** Don't challenge your sleeve.
- **You must maintain your intake of protein** to avoid malnutrition and maintain muscle mass, and avoid serious complications related to low protein levels in your body.
- **You should be maintaining a diet with 65+ grams of protein a day and 2 quarts of liquids per day.** The total daily calories will vary between 800-1000, depending on your weight at one year. We caution patients to not exceed 1000-1200 calories per day, unless we advise you otherwise. Patients who go below their ideal weight will need to eat more, especially carbohydrates, to maintain their weight.
- **Keep in mind that the stomach pouch will**

only accommodate approximately 4 oz (½ cup). Use small plates or food scales to guide your estimation of how much your stomach can hold at any one time. The starting volume of your stomach does not necessarily correlate with the volume of food you can have at one sitting. The stomach can be quite contracted or irritable and only allow a fraction of the total volume in. You should never put more than 3-4 oz of food on your plate at one time. Write down what you are eating and when. Until your eye is really trained to gauge how much you are consuming, you may be overdoing it. Even still, your eyes may be bigger than your stomach . . . measure out your portions to be on the safe side.

Head hunger

As you probably know, the contribution of "stress eating" or "head hunger" to morbid obesity cannot be overemphasized. Some patients have discussed these issues with psychologists and therapists throughout many years of their adult life. Occasionally, after months of following a stricter diet after surgery, older habits and "stress eating" behaviors can slowly become a problem. Most patients can say that even after 1-2 years after surgery, they are only able to eat 1-2 small bites of well chewed chicken. However, they can eat many more French fries, potato chips, nuts, beans, etc.—all the foods that would sabotage good weight loss and lead to significant weight regain. Even if the surgical procedure has gone well, there are still psychological issues that can cause failure and must be addressed. In these cases, we often advise our patients to seek psychological or even psychiatric help after surgery to help with these issues. Substituting physical activities and hobbies are common solutions to these problems. Cancel lunch meetings and plan walking dates! Plenty of patients are bike-riding, hiking, swimming, running, and enjoying other activities with friends and family. The difference after surgery is that most patients are now satisfied with small quantities of solid protein-rich foods, and thus the hunger factor is diminished in contributing to the problems.

Concentrated sweets

Most of the following foods and beverages are filled with "empty" calories in the form of sugar. Sugar-free versions of these items are acceptable. These products provide mainly calories with limited nutritional value (that is, small amounts of vitamins, minerals, protein, and fiber).

Every bite counts after weight loss surgery. An adequate amount of protein needs to be consumed to prevent malnutrition secondary to mal-absorption following surgery. Filling up on these "concentrated sweets" can prevent weight loss and can replace healthier foods from your diet. They actually don't help you feel full. If you choose to eat healthier, more nutritional foods first with each meal, you will more likely not have any room or appetite for nutritionally "empty" foods.

Foods to avoid

- Ice cream and frozen treats (unless sugar-free/fat-free)
- Soft drinks
- Chocolate milk or flavored milk products
- Lemonade
- Pudding and custard - (unless sugar free and low-fat)
- Kool Aid®
- Sweetened, added-fruit, or frozen yogurt
- Sugared ice tea

- Dried fruits - high sugar content
- Fruit juices and fruit drinks
- Canned or frozen fruits in syrup - high sugar content
- Table sugar (Splenda® okay in small amounts)
- Jellies, jams and preserves
- Honey, molasses
- Sugar-coated cereals
- Candy
- Doughnuts and pastries
- Regular Jell-O®
- Popsicles®
- Regular gum
- Cakes
- Pies
- Maple syrup
- Cookies
- Sherbet/sorbet/gelato

More on carbohydrates

Low fiber ("white") starches and simple sugars are very easy to overeat, which is one reason people consume too many calories and gain weight. Managing carbohydrate intake is essential in order to meet restricted calorie goals for weight loss. Being aware of hidden sources and added calories in the carbohydrates we eat is also very important. Splenda® is a sugar substitute and okay in small amounts. Some nutritionists feel that Splenda® may cause sugar cravings in patients after weight loss surgery. Also, Splenda® can cause diarrhea in some individuals. Saccharin® or Aspartame® may be better if you require a sweetener; again, consume in small amounts.

Starchy foods include breads, cereals, grains, noodles, rice, starchy vegetables, baked goods, snack foods, and crackers. Many starchy foods may be low-fat or fat-free but can contain hidden sugars. Many have hidden fats added for the cooking or baking process and for added flavor and appeal. High-fat and sugar-loaded starchy foods include baked goods (cookies, cakes, etc.), some cereals, breakfast and energy bars, chips, and other snack foods.

If you must eat starches, again opt for the more whole grains, not empty calories with no nutritional value. Read your labels. Fats are often added unknowingly to low-fat, starchy foods, which adds additional unaccountable calories. Examples are butter on toast, mayonnaise on a sandwich, cream sauce on noodles, cream cheese on bagels, and sour cream on potatoes. We all love the taste of these combinations but can learn to enjoy the taste of food instead of the high-calorie additions. Using very little or a lower fat/non-fat substitute is also an option.

Review the portion sizes of the foods in the starch group so you can limit your total carbohydrate intake when meal planning. Avoid simple sugars, and be aware of added/hidden sugars and fats in your favorite foods and the fats you add to your carbohydrates. This will help to keep calorie levels lower to aid in permanent weight loss after surgery. If the packaging states that a food item is fat free, you can be certain it is loaded with carbohydrates. If it states that the item is sugar free, you can be certain it is loaded with fat. When in doubt, look at the total calories. If the calorie count is very low, it will probably be okay to eat. Read labels!

Remember, to maximize weight loss the following should be avoided:

- Peanut butter
- Nuts
- Sausage
- Hot dogs
- Bratwurst
- Bologna
- Salami
- Breaded & fried foods
- Fast food
- Rice
- Pasta
- Desserts
- Potato chips/pretzels
- Popcorn
- Alcohol
- Candy, cakes, cookies, ice cream (including sugar free)
- Heavy sauces & gravy (i.e. Alfredo)
- Fruit Juice

Chapter 7

Exercise and Your Gastric Sleeve

The importance of exercise

The most successful patients (in terms of overall health and weight loss) who have had the gastric sleeve procedure have two things in common:

(1) They follow their dietary recommendations closely, and

(2) they initiate and maintain a regular exercise program.

It is essential that, within the first four weeks after surgery, you begin a regular exercise program. Initially, this may simply be walking around the neighborhood, five times per week for 40-60 minutes each time. Later (three to four months post-op), it will also involve low-impact resistance training (swimming, light weight-lifting, rowing, etc.). This will guarantee not only a good weight loss, but will also improve your stamina, energy level, and overall health. Remember, you lose weight when the energy expenditure is greater than the amount of calories (energy) eaten. Studies have consistently shown that individuals who make a habit of regular exercise not only live longer and have fewer health problems, but are able to maintain their weight loss indefinitely. Always try to choose activities that are affordable and that you enjoy. In doing so, you will give yourself the best chance at maintaining a healthy lifestyle.

I recommend you start slow with exercise. Don't try to overdo it when you start. Remember that the key is consistency and not trying to kill yourself with the exercise. Try to start walking 7 days after surgery by doing 15 to 20 minutes on a treadmill. Plan to do exercise in an air -conditioned facility to avoid too much sun exposure and dehydration. Keep this rhythm, doing the walking 4 times per week. After you're 15 days out of surgery, you may increase the walking time to 30 to 40 minutes per session.

There are many reasons for starting your own walking

program. Here are just a few:

- Improved quality of life
- Improved muscle strength
- Relieved pain
- Increased concentration at work
- Getting in touch with nature
- Increased blood flow
- Feeling better about yourself
- Stress reduction
- Weight loss
- Meeting your neighbors
- Exercising your dog; he'll love you for it.

We don't recommend intense exercise like ab crunches or weight-lifting until you're 30 days out. The main reason is that one of your incisions (the largest one) where your resected stomach is taken out is closed using a non-absorbable suture to prevent a hernia in the long run. This heals in 30 days. If you do some sort of extreme exercise you may pop this inner stitch and the risk of a hernia can elevate. So keep it moderate for the first 30 days.

Swimming

Some people like swimming as a cardio exercise. It actually is great! Just try not to submerge yourself in water for the first 15 days after surgery. Wait until your wounds are completely healed so you don't have to worry about a wound infection. After 15 days you're good to go with the swimming or taking a bath in a tub.

"A successful surgery does not make a successful patient." Your surgeon can only do his part in your success; the rest is up to you.

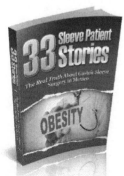

Chapter 8

Common Complaints, Risks, and Complications

Wound care

In general, surgeons apply Steri-strips™ over your incisions, which will generally fall off within a week or so; please don't pick or peel them off sooner. Picking them off prematurely may cause the wound to open up. Showering is permitted after 24 hours post-op, but stand with your back to the water so shower isn't directly hitting incisions. You may take a bath after two weeks if all your incisions are healed. You may also notice some bruising around your incisions; this is normal. Occasionally, and unavoidable during surgery, a small vessel maybe hit with one of the trocars, causing a small bleed that can result in a large discoloration. This will disappear over time and is nothing to be overly concerned about. If you experience increasing redness, pain, or warmth at any of the wounds, you may have an infection, so please contact your surgeon's office. A small amount of redness (less than ½ inch) is common and usually consistent with healing. Some patients may have a small amount of drainage from their wounds. The body fills the open space beneath wounds with fluid, and this tends to drain out. It is inconvenient and you may need to use a couple of gauze pads each day to catch the fluid. If the drainage increases in volume and saturates several gauze pads each day, or becomes thick and foul-smelling, again, contact your doctor as there may be a need to be seen either by your surgeon or your primary care provider. The largest of your incisions (usually on the left-hand side) is normally closed with a tighter suture, so you may feel a tugging, tightness, pull, pinching, or burning sensation. This is all normal and will resolve as the suture itself dissolves and the swelling disappears.

Leaks

A leak is a hole from the stomach or intestines that goes directly into the abdominal cavity. If it's going to occur, it is usually within the first 2 weeks after surgery and must be diagnosed and treated immediately. To repair it usually requires an additional surgery and an extended hospital stay. You do not want to have this happen to you. This is the main reason for the postoperative diet, which consists of liquids. Why liquids? Liquids move much more smoothly through the sleeve without causing tension or stress on the recently stapled or stapled/sutured stomach. If you were to eat something that is not liquid in the first weeks, it would cause tension or pressure and could favor the development of a leak. The doctor's experience and technique, plus the fact you are drinking liquids only the first 3 weeks lowers the possibility of this complication. It often occurs more frequently in patients undergoing a revision surgery (example: switching from a LAP-BAND® to a Gastric Sleeve), meaning they had a previous stomach or weight loss procedure, which makes the surgery more difficult due to scar tissue or adhesions. The following signs may indicate a leak: increasing abdominal pain, fevers, sweats, difficulty breathing, rapid heartbeat, chills, and an elevation in your white blood cell count. If any of these happen while still in the hospital, you will be immediately taken care of. If you have already been discharged to your home, it is very important to notify your surgeon as soon as possible if you are having any of the above symptoms. Diagnosis of a leak can be confirmed with an X-ray test with a contrast material or a CT scan. Surgery is almost always the next step to repair this serious problem. Do not hesitate to call with any questions if you are concerned.

Gas pain or discomfort

This is commonly misunderstood because there are actually two types of gas discomfort that may appear in the immediate postoperative period. The first type that I will explain is very uncommon, and, if present, usually lasts between a couple of hours to 6-12 hours after the surgery. This type of gas pain is due to the gas insufflated into your abdomen to create a cavity during the surgery. This means that any laparoscopic procedure involves CO_2 gas to be insufflated into your tummy. This will help visualize the abdominal organs once the tiny camera (laparoscope) goes into your belly. If the physician were to position this camera without insufflating the CO_2 gas, he or she most likely wouldn't be able to distinguish the organs inside the abdomen. Right after surgery this gas is released from the stomach, but in some cases a small percentage of this gas may be left in the abdomen because it may "hide" in between the organs, intestines, etc. If this is the case, once the patient starts to move a bit in the recovery room or back in his/her room, this gas tends to elevate and may lie just underneath the diaphragm. This will irritate a nerve called the Phrenic, which will cause a referred pain to the left upper shoulder. This pain may last up to 6 to 12 hours if present and is very well tolerated with mild medication for pain.

The second type of gas pain is caused because of the size of your new sleeved stomach. This means that because you now have a "new" stomach with a different shape that can hold only small amounts of food, it also can hold only very small amounts of air or gas. In other words, everybody has air or gas in the stomach, but in a regular stomach, when air gets to a certain point you can actually burp out this air. Now, with your new stomach, you may have difficulty the first few days managing this air. So if air sits in your sleeve it may cause some discomfort. I usually tell my patients that a good example to understand this would be to compare the new sleeved stomach to a baby's stomach. Newborn babies have a hard time managing air in their stomachs. So parents are instructed that after the baby is fed they do some patting on the baby's back. This will eventually cause the baby to burp. This air that is burped is actually air that the baby swallowed during the feeding and will stay in the stomach. If not released, the baby may cry or have some discomfort. This is why baby feeding bottles have a special tip to help the baby swallow less air.

The same is applicable to patients with a gastric sleeve during the first few days, and this is why the use of straws is not recommended in the first few weeks after the surgery. If you use a straw to sip liquids down, you will put larger amounts of air in your new stomach, causing discomfort. When you suck on a straw, you first draw a column of air followed by the liquid you will ingest. So drinking from a glass directly or using sport bottle caps will prevent this.

Managing this type of gas discomfort is relatively simple. Although you can get somebody to pat your back until you burp, we recommend you walk! This is the best medication the first couple of days after surgery. The reason is that the walking will cause the small amounts of air or gas that build up in your stomach or that you swallowed to either pass to your intestine or come up as a burp. Either way, the air will move from your recently operated stomach and will cause relief. So, as I tell my patients, "The more walking you do the better you feel!"

IV site discomfort

This is a very common complaint. It is possible during your hospital stay that your IV may become infiltrated. This happens at times when the vein simply cannot handle the amount of fluids passed through it. When this happens the fluids will leak outside the vein and into your tissues. It may cause a large lump or goose egg and may be tender, warm, or hard to the touch. If this does happen, please use warm compresses for several days (20 min. on, 20 min. off) to help the fluids absorb. You may take Tylenol® for the discomfort as well. Don't be alarmed if this takes a few days to a couple of weeks to completely resolve itself. It you are overly concerned or have a question, please don't hesitate to contact your doctor's office.

Nausea and vomiting

Some patients have mild nausea in the first few months following the gastric sleeve procedure. Nausea can be treated in several ways. First, try some decaffeinated green tea. This can be very effective. If the nausea is more than just mild, I recommend you contact your surgeon's office. We surgeons will want to know about this and may need to prescribe a medication to help. If the nausea persists, this may be a sign of a problem and, therefore, we should know about it. Both nausea and vomiting may occur after eating too fast, drinking liquids while eating, not chewing enough, or eating more than the stomach can comfortably hold. It is necessary to learn to eat very slowly and chew foods thoroughly. If vomiting occurs, stop drinking or eating until the nausea passes. After the nausea subsides, resume only fluid intake for 12-24 hours before attempting to eat solid foods. Nausea and vomiting can also be triggered by trying new foods. If this happens, allow a few days to pass before trying the same food again. Repetitive vomiting to the point that liquids cannot be kept down is potentially dangerous. Again, contact your doctor if the vomiting becomes a problem.

Heartburn

Acid reflux symptoms may worsen initially after the restrictive gastric sleeve procedure because of delayed stomach emptying. If you do have symptoms of heartburn, eating or drinking too quickly may also cause it. It may also be caused by stomach spasms or a stricture. Please contact your doctor's office if you are having troubles with heartburn or regurgitation, as it can be a sign of a problem and we may need to start you on some over-the-counter or prescription medication. Don't wait more than a day or two to call if you are having this problem. You can purchase some Prilosec® OTC or Zantac® 150 mg just to have on hand in case this problem continues after you finish the medication the doctor gives you on discharge.

Stool frequency and diarrhea

You may have loose, frequent stools for a few weeks or even months after surgery. Remember that in the initial weeks you will not be having any solid food, and since only liquids are in your GI track this may result in loose stools. This condition is something we see often in Gastric Sleeve patients. This will slowly improve as you modify your diet. If this is problematic, please notify your doctor and he or she can prescribe a medication to address this problem. Avoid those foods that seem to cause you to have diarrhea. You may wish to use a stool softener on a daily basis as your consumption of food has decreased as has the amount of your fiber intake. You may take an occasional over-the-counter medication, such as Kaopectate® (for diarrhea) or Dulcolax® Tablets (for constipation) to help with bowel problems. However, you should **not** take drugs such as Imodium® or Ex-Lax® unless you have spoken with your doctor first. Also, as a rule of thumb, if you have diarrhea while on protein drinks, then change to a different kind. If you have constipation, drink more liquids. If you continue to have an issue with constipation, you may use a daily stool softener once or twice a day.

Hair loss

You may or may not experience hair loss; hair may possibly come out in clumps while brushing. (Normal hair loss is 75-100 hairs per day). Do not fret, since this is common with rapid weight loss by any method. Hair loss will slow and stop as you approach your goal weight and your weight loss slows. At that point, your hair will begin to grow back with finer hair. We may order blood tests if we are concerned about malnutrition causing hair loss. However, most of the time, the hair loss is a result of hormonal changes from changes in fat cells.

Some patients find that taking a hair and nail supplement that can be purchased from GNC® or other vitamin shop can be helpful. Another option is to take the following supplements, which may also help prevent or slow hair loss:

- Co-Enzyme Q/10: 25-50mg per day
- Biotin: 300mcg per day
- Flax Seed Oil: 1-2 grams per day, gel-tabs, oil or sprinkles
- Zinc: 50mg per day

Remember, there are no bald weight loss patients. All the hair that you lose should re-grow once you have reached your goal weight.

The length of the incision

This is one example when "smaller is better." The larger or longer the incision, the more likely that a hernia will develop. After most abdominal surgeries that are performed in an open or traditional manner (as opposed to laparoscopically), the likelihood of a hernia occurring is about 10%. This number may go as high as 30-40% in patients who are very obese or malnourished. When a surgery is performed laparoscopically (surgery using small instruments and a camera) through very small incisions (usually less than ½ inch), the likelihood of a hernia occurring drops to less than 1%. This is one of the real advantages of laparoscopic surgery over open or conventional surgery—one that has been proven in many medical studies over and over again. However, if you feel a lump under one or more of the incisions (especially the bigger incisions) in the next 2-4 weeks after the surgery, it does not necessarily mean it is a hernia. It may even be a bit tender, but remember that there is inflammation tissue and a scar is forming under each incision too. This thick, dense tissue will become softer 6-8 weeks after surgery.

Tenderness on the larger incision

The one larger incision (normally on the left side of your abdomen) is located where the residual portion of stomach had been removed. This may be more tender and painful for a while, especially when moving or turning. It has been sutured tighter than the rest to prevent a possible hernia from developing. This incision could be closed with an absorbable or non-absorbable suture, depending on the surgeon's preference.

So, if you feel a sharp pain, pull, tug, burn, sting, pinch, tingle, that is all normal and you should not become alarmed . . . it will resolve over time. Sometimes a heating pad on low will help to resolve this discomfort as well. If you are in severe discomfort you should contact your surgeon.

Pulmonary Embolism

A pulmonary embolism, or PE, is a blood clot that travels from elsewhere in the body, usually the legs and pelvis, to the arteries in the lungs. The resultant effect on the body can be just some difficulty breathing but can also cause shortness of breath, fast heart rate, heart attack, and death. A PE usually starts as a blood clot forming in the leg but can move to the lungs unexpectedly. Leg pain may be one of the first symptoms of a problem. The risk of a fatal PE is relatively low. Risk factors for PE include obesity, smoking, undergoing major surgery, cancer, oral contraceptives, age > 40, trauma, pregnancy, having a heart attack or heart failure, having a stroke, varicose veins, prior blood clot problems, and underlying "hyper-clotting" disorder.

We as surgeons help minimize the chance of a deep vein thrombosis and a PE by implementing several methods like wrapping your legs tightly with a stretch bandage, using a special air-compression device during surgery to keep the blood moving in your legs during the operation, and using low molecular weight heparin or similar medications. It is important for you to know that walking soon after the operation is over is very beneficial too. While you are in bed after surgery, it is good to exercise pumping your calf muscles to keep the flow of blood moving. Walking every day while you are awake helps significantly, especially while you are in the hospital.

This activity should be continued at home.

Maintenance of the gastric sleeve

The gastric sleeve procedure differs from LAP -BAND® surgery because it is free of "maintenance." Meaning you will not need any band adjustments or "fills," nor will you have any erosion or slippage because you have no band. The gastric sleeve is a procedure that requires less "maintenance" than malabsorption procedures like the gastric bypass (Roux-en-Y) or the duodenal switch but still requires you to take care of your sleeve and your body. We recommend annual lab testing to all patients having the gastric sleeve surgery even though patients are free of any symptoms. These labs will check for anemia, blood glucose, liver, iron levels, and evidence of vitamin deficiency, among other things. This will help us to evaluate your nutritional condition and see if you need to make some changes in your diet or supplements. For the lab testing, please remember to avoid all vitamin supplements for 3 days prior to lab draw and have tests obtained while fasting (no food or drink for 12 hours prior).

Recommended post-op lab testing

The annual post-op lab testing that we recommend is ICD-9 (Diagnosis Code for insurance billing: 783.12)

- CBC
- Pro-time, INR, PTT
- Iron, Total Binding Capacity, Ferritin, Transferrin

- Comprehensive Metabolic Panel
- Carnitine, Folate, Vitamin A, Vitamin B-6, Vitamin B-12, Vitamin D, Zinc
- Lipid Panel: Triglycerides, LDL, VLDL, HDL, Cholesterol Total

Chapter 9

Frequently Asked Questions

I wanted to provide this special section that would make my book unique in the gastric sleeve realm. I've placed a list of the most frequently asked questions here. The possibilities of questions on this subject are endless so I wanted to make this more fun with interaction with you. If you want a question answered, send it over via my social media networks and post your question. This way the database for questions will grow and this will help clear more doubts of future patients too.

Preoperative Questions

1. This is my last resort; what if this doesn't work for me? You will lose weight with the gastric sleeve procedure. All you need to do is follow the guidelines given by your surgeon. Follow them as they are the best route to achieve your goals. By doing this you will lose the amount of weight required to make you healthier and live life to the fullest. It will work!

2. How much will I lose?

This depends mainly on the patient, but it also depends on the surgeon's technique. You will lose between 65-90% of your excess body weight. Therefore, the heavier the patient is the more amount of weight in pounds he/she will lose.

3. Does having the gastric sleeve guarantee rapid weight loss?

On all the weight loss surgery procedures, the objective is to lose more weight than dieting and/or exercising alone. The weight loss with the gastric sleeve is similar in general to a gastric bypass surgery but faster than an adjustable gastric band. The weight loss depends greatly on every patient but on average it is steady and progressive. The more the patient weighs prior to surgery, the more he/she has to lose, so weight loss will be faster. On average, a patient with a gastric sleeve may lose between 2-4 lbs per week. There may be periods when the weight loss may stall. These stalls are normal and give the body a chance to "adapt" to its new weight.

Normally, this is the phase where the patients lose more sizes in clothing.

4. Can I convert my gastric sleeve into another procedure down the road?

Yes, the sleeve gives the patient the option to convert to either a gastric bypass or a duodenal switch. These two procedures are mal-absorption surgeries that involve re-routing intestines and are more prone to vitamin deficiencies than a purely restrictive procedure like the sleeve. Studies have shown that a conversion to another procedure, also called revision, is more likely in high-BMI (Body Mass Index) patients >50 or when a larger sleeve or stomach using a larger bougie was done in the initial surgery.

5. Will my hair fall out?

This may or may not happen since this is related to weight loss surgery, but this may be more intense if you fill up your sleeve with bad quality food that contains little or no needed nutrients. Since patients have a very small stomach capacity, if they eat something non-nutritious, by the time they want to sit down and eat something more healthy, they will not be able to since the sleeve is already full. If the hair does start to fall, it is recommended to take supplements to help stop the hair loss and it will help with the re-growth of it. See more on hair loss in the Common Complaints section of this book.

6. What can I do to improve my fitness for surgery ahead of time?

Cardiovascular exercise and blowing up regular balloons (10-20 balloons per day) will help in getting you in condition for surgery.

7. Will I need to stop taking medication before surgery? How soon?

No, you don't need to stop your medication except for certain NSAIDS (Advil®, Motrin®, Naproxen®, etc.), aspirin, Plavix®, among other medications. Please check with your doctor since he/ she will let you know what you need to stop prior to surgery and for how long, if applicable.

8. Can I take vitamins until surgery?

Yes, taking vitamins does not interfere at all with surgery.

9. Do I have to do anything special the last few days before surgery, such as a clear diet, fasting, or laxatives?

The only thing necessary for a gastric sleeve surgery is to fast for 8 hrs. at least. There is no need for colon-cleansing, laxatives, etc.

10. What kinds of things could prevent/delay the surgery? There may be several reasons that may delay surgery, like abnormal laboratory findings in your blood work that can make the surgery risky or unsafe. Also, a severe upper airway infection can cause a delay to your surgery due to mucus and secretions, which can give your anesthesiologist a difficult time dealing with your intubation and maintaining a secure airway during surgery. For this reason, it may be appropriate to delay the surgery until the infection has subsided.

11. Can I get pregnant after the sleeve procedure?

Yes! Many OB/GYN doctors refer patients who are seeking to get pregnant but can't due to their obesity or to polycystic ovarian syndrome (PCOS). After having the gastric sleeve procedure, the PCOS is reversed in the vast majority of the cases, and patients are able to get pregnant and have regular menstrual cycles. I don't recommend getting pregnant in the first 12 months post-op even though I've seen patients who have done it. Take your maternal vitamins and supplements and everything should progress as a normal pregnancy.

12. Am I too old or too young for the gastric sleeve surgery? General guidelines by the American Society for Metabolic and Bariatric Surgery (ASMBS) state that patients should be between the ages of 18-64 to have weight loss surgery, but we have seen more and more younger teenagers experience amazing results, as have patients over the age of 64. This is a guideline but not a rule, and the bariatric surgeon will analyze each case individually.

Hospital Stay Questions

1. What is a "bougie"?

A bougie is a term given to a calibration tube. The surgeon, while performing the gastric sleeve, normally uses this calibration tube. While the patient is under anesthesia and during the procedure, a tube or bougie is inserted through the mouth, down the esophagus and into the stomach. This bougie has a certain diameter or size. The size is expressed in "French" or "Fr." This measuring unit is commonly used in medicine with catheters, drains, etc.1 inch = 76.2 French, 1 French = 0.333 millimeters. This bougie is used as a pattern to cut enough stomach so the patient has the most amount of weight loss possible while leaving enough stomach behind for the patient's nutrition needs. After finishing the gastric sleeve procedure and prior to bringing the patient back from the anesthesia, the anesthesiologist removes the bougie from the patient's mouth.

2. How are the incisions closed? Staples? Stitches? Over sew?

This varies from surgeon to surgeon, but in the vast majority of the cases we close the incisions with subdermal stitches (underneath the skin) with absorbable material then place some Steristrips®. These stitches self-dissolve, making the incisions almost care-free.

3. Do you automatically remove the gallbladder and/or appendix?

There is no indication to remove the gallbladder or any other organ at the time of surgery unless there is a specific reason to do so. If you have gallstones at the time of surgery then you may undergo sleeve surgery and have your gallbladder removed at the same time, otherwise it is not recommended.

4. Where will the incisions be made?

The number of incisions and where they are placed will depend on your surgeon's technique. The procedure is normally done with 5 or 6 small incisions. Here is a

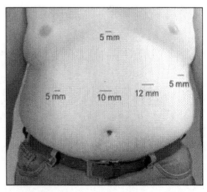

diagram of where we place our incisions.

5. How long will I be in surgery?

This depends on several factors like your body mass index (BMI) and your surgeon and his team. Patients with a BMI under 45 in general undergo much simpler surgeries than higher BMI patients due to more visceral fat, which is accumulated fat around the organs inside your abdomen, giving less space to work in. Currently in our practice our average time to complete a gastric sleeve surgery is about 35 minutes. Higher BMI patients or more complex scenarios can take up to an hour.

6. Will I have a nasogastric tube when I come out of surgery?

No, there is no need for the use of a nasogastric tube.

7. Will I have an epidural?

No, you will not have an epidural; all weight loss surgery procedures done through laparoscopy are done under general anesthesia and do not require an epidural.

8. Will I be in ICU (intensive care unit)?

No, unless there are important pre-existing conditions

that require the support of an intensive care unit. About 99% of our patients will not need the ICU.

9. Will I have IVs?

We use one IV line for a time period of 24 hours once you start taking some ice chips. After that time we position a heparin lock to have the vein accessible in case we need it, but if there is no need of having it (no nausea or pain) it will be taken out completely.

10. Will I be on a ventilator?

Not after surgery unless an important preexisting condition obligates the use of an intensive care unit. Undergoing general anesthesia mandates the use of a ventilator during surgery only but not post-op.

11. Do you insert a urinary catheter?

No, since the surgery is generally under an hour, there is no need for a catheter. We do encourage the patients to empty their bladder prior to going into the operating room.

12. Will I have drainage tubes after surgery?

We normally don't place drains in sleeves as a primary

procedure. We only place drains in some revision surgeries from LAP-BAND®s to sleeves. This varies from surgeon to surgeon. It is a controversial subject among bariatric surgeons.

13. Will I need a binder after surgery?

There is no need for any special garments or binders after laparoscopic surgery.

14. How soon will I be allowed to consume ice chips after the surgery?

In our practice you will be able to start with ice after24 hours of having surgery. This may vary from surgeon to surgeon. The ice has two main functions: (1) It will help you keep hydrated and (2) The cold of the ice will help reduce the swollen tissue from the surgery. This helps greatly when done prior to the leak test to have a better picture and visualization of the new sleeve.

15. How soon will I be allowed to consume ice water?

After you start consuming ice chips for some hours we do a leak test to verify everything is good. Depending on how much swollen tissue we see on the test we will permit you to start sipping water. This is usually about 36 hours post-op.

16. How soon and how often should I walk after the surgery? Usually patients start getting up to the restroom 2-3 hours after surgery and doing some walking in their room. After 24 hours, we make patients walk the hospital halls 2 or 3 laps every 30 minutes or so. You need to keep in mind that walking is the best "medication," and the more walking you do, the better you'll feel.

17. How long is the hospital stay?
Depending on your surgeon's program, the average stay for a gastric sleeve surgery in the hospital is 48 hours.

18. Am I required to stay in the hospital until I have a bowel movement?
This is not necessary; remember that some people follow a liquid diet prior to surgery, then after surgery you continue with a liquid diet and there is nothing solid in your intestines, so a bowel movement may take a few days. It is

not necessary in order for you to be discharged from the hospital.

19. Are there any reasons why the procedure may not be performed once I am in surgery?

Since we do the surgery through laparoscopy, we get to place a tiny camera inside to visualize your abdominal cavity. Possibly the biggest issue can be encountering a huge liver (officially called non-alcoholic fatty liver disease), which won't give us good visualization of the stomach and reduces the space in which we can work to carry out the surgery. This is related to not being compliant with the pre- op diet. There are other reasons that may contribute to aborting the gastric sleeve surgery, such as finding a tumor, but these are conditions that are very rare.

20. Will I vomit a lot?

One of people's greatest fears is vomiting after a surgery involving the stomach. Nowadays, we have some amazingly efficient medications to prevent nausea. In our practice, we strongly believe in making the patient's recovery the easiest possible, so anti-nausea medication is already scheduled out during the patient's stay, resulting in a nausea-free surgery in the vast majority of patients.

Postoperative Questions

1. How does my body know when to stop losing weight? The gastric sleeve is very different regarding losing too much weight compared to the gastric bypass or the duodenal switch. These surgeries can cause you to lose too much weight or have a difficult time maintaining because they have the intestinal component, which prevents the patient from absorbing 100% of the nutrients eaten. The gastric sleeve procedure will only do so much for you. In other words, you also have to exert some effort to achieve your goal. As I explained on the previous question, the procedure will leave you with some extra pounds. In other words, the surgery will not make you lose too much weight.

2. How much will my sleeve stretch out? Depending on what size of bougie or calibration tube your surgeon used in the procedure is how much your sleeve will stretch out with time. In other words, the bigger the calibration tube or bougie, the more "stretchy" stomach is left in you. This will result in more capacity of your stomach with time. What studies have shown is that if you use a 32 Fr bougie you will have excellent weight loss without going so small in size that it can cause you trouble like strictures or narrowing in your sleeve. If a 32 Fr bougie is used, the sleeve will stretch out a minimum percentage with time, and will never stretch out to the size the stomach was before surgery. Commonly used bougies for the gastric sleeve surgery can range between 28-60 Fr.

3. Will I have to diet forever after surgery?

No. Patients who have had a gastric sleeve procedure pretty much eat anything they desire; what changes is the capacity of the stomach. Unlike other bariatric procedures like the adjustable gastric band, after which patients very often feel sick and vomit frequently during their post -operative life and have to stay away from certain foods like meat or bread, the gastric sleeve does not create these problems.

4. What is the percentage of proteins, carbohydrates, and fat I have to look out for after surgery?

These percentages pretty much stay the same as prior

to having the surgery. From 45 to 65% of the calorie intake should come from carbohydrates, 20-35% from fat, and 10-35% from protein. Postoperative patients should focus on eating the protein first always. The reason is that while the patient is losing weight, we focus on trying to lose weight from fat tissue and not from muscle. So don't fill up your sleeve with carbohydrates or fat; fill it up with proteins to maintain your muscle tissue and lose the weight from stored fat.

5. How many grams of protein do I have to consume daily?

The current recommendation for protein intake in adults is0.8 g of protein per kilogram of ideal body weight per day. This means that if your ideal body weight is around 70 kg (154 lbs) you should consume close to 56 g of protein per day.

6. Will I be able to drink alcohol after I have my surgery?

Drinking alcohol after a bariatric procedure is not recommended because alcohol will take longer to metabolize in the patient's body; therefore, serum levels of alcohol will rise more quickly and will be maintained longer in a bariatric patient. When patients insist on wanting to drink, I recommend drinking very small amounts of alcohol once their weight has become stable or they have reached their goal weight (after 12-18 months). I still warn them that they stand the risk of getting drunk with small amounts of alcohol and may take longer to become sober.

7. Why are fluids so important?

Fluids are very important from the very first day you start the liquid diet right after surgery. The first 3-4 days after starting the liquid diet patients may have a hard time getting enough liquids in because the sleeve may be very swollen.

This is normal since the surgery was done only a few days ago. As the swollen tissue starts to subside, the patient needs to learn a trick to have a good daily fluid intake. The best way to have good fluid intake is by having a bottle of water, tea, Gatorade®, Cristal Light®, etc. in your hand at all times while you are awake. You should take a small sip and wait 2-3 minutes. After this you will be able to sip again. While doing this you are giving enough time for the liquid you ingested to go through your sleeve and pass to your intestines. If you ingest liquids more frequently than every 2-3 minutes or you gulp liquids down, what you will experience is an uncomfortable sensation caused by the column of liquid "stacked up" in your sleeved stomach. This also can be followed by nausea and/or cramping. The other thing patients must avoid is drinking liquids out of straws. The reason is that when we drink out of straws we intake a column of air prior to the liquid reaching the mouth. This air may reach your new stomach and may produce an uncomfortable sensation too, like bloating, nausea, cramping, etc. I suggest drinking out of a glass directly or from sport bottle caps that are specifically designed to prevent athletes from taking in air while drinking water. You should focus on taking in 64 oz (2 liters) of liquids daily. The only way to know if you are taking enough fluids daily is by measuring them. This way you will know that if you are not drinking enough liquids you need to push it a little harder to reach your daily goal. Also, it is important to stay away from the heat. I always tell my patients to stay in air-conditioned facilities, especially the first week. If patients would like to enjoy being outside, they can do so only if it's cool or by waiting until dusk. Transpiration or sweating can be a very important cause of dehydration in recently operated patients, especially if they are only ingesting the minimum daily requirement.

8. Will I be constipated after surgery?

Normally there is no change in the patient's intestinal habits. But in the initial phase of the liquid diet, patients may experience loose stools or a decrease in the frequency of bowel movements. The main reason patients have loose stools is because they are only taking liquids in their diets. Since no solid food is in the intestinal track, there is nothing to give shape or form to the stools, so they are also in liquid state. This same reason of ingesting only liquids may also cause some patients to have a decrease in bowel movements. If the patient experiences constipation after he or she starts eating solids, one of the more frequent causes is dehydration or a lack of liquid intake. This is another reason why a patient should keep track of how much liquid is taken.

9. Should I take vitamins and which ones?

This was something that was in debate years ago when we started doing the sleeve. The answer nowadays is "yes," you should take vitamins, especially during the first 8-12 months after surgery. This is the period where you lose the most amount of weight, and taking supplements helps your body have all the nutrients you need even if you don't eat that much. I recommend my patients to take either the chewable multivitamins or the liquid form. It is also recommended for the patient to take vitamin B12 and calcium/vitamin D complex too. For more information on this subject, please go over the Vitamins section of this book.

10. Will my sleeve "blow up" in an airplane?

No. Remember that your sleeve will act as a regular stomach. The only thing that changes after surgery is your stomach capacity and your hunger sensation; both will be much less.

11. When can I resume having sex?

Whenever the patient feels good about it. It is very important that the patient understands that having sex will not cause the sleeve to burst, or a staple to pop, nor will it cause the sleeve to leak. Having sex does not interfere at all with the sleeve. So as soon as the patient feels good about having sex, he or she can resume sexual activity.

12. Will the staples of the sleeve sound off the alarms at airports?

No. The amount of titanium of the micro staples is so small that it is undetectable by metal detectors at airports. Anyway, we strongly advise patients to have an ID card or medical alert tag whenever they travel, as well as the numbers to their doctor's office.

13. Will the staples dissolve or will they stay in the body forever?

The staples are titanium made. They will not dissolve ever, but the patients must understand that the function of the staples is to hold the stomach together while it heals(15-21 days). After this period, the staples will stay in the same place they were placed during the surgery. These staples are 100% biocompatible and will not cause the patient any issues for the rest of his/her life.

14. Can I have MRI's (Magnetic Resonance Imaging) after surgery because of the titanium staples?

Yes, you can have MRIs after surgery, although there are some experts in radiology who recommend you

wait2 months after surgery to do this type of study.
After this time it is totally safe to do this type of test
since the amount of titanium you carry with you is so
small and your stomach is completely healed.

15. Can I get a leak 1 year out?

No. The risk of a leak is greater during the first few
hours or days of the surgery. After the healing process
of the sleeve is over, the risk of a leak is zero, although
any patient, even prior to gastric sleeve surgery can
develop an ulcer, which is different from a leak.

16. How do you get tested for a leak after surgery?

One of the simplest ways to do this is to do an X-ray
study with a fluoroscopy machine. This machine gives a
continuous X-ray vision while the patient ingests a
special contrast material. This material is easily viewed
and can be followed through its path along the sleeve.
If there were to be a leak it is usually seen as liquid that
does not follow the normal path it should.

There are other methods to check for a leak like a CT
(Computed Tomography)scan. This method introduces
the patient into a machine that with the use of X-rays

will determine the actual anatomy of the patient's stomach. Oral contrast material is usually used too.

17. Why is protein so important?

Protein is very important because if patients are not careful they may not get enough and may start losing weight off the body's muscle tissue. This is simple to understand since the body is losing weight because it has a low calorie intake. What the patients want is to lose weight off the stored fat tissue— not the muscle. So what the patients need to do is ingest enough protein, and the way to do this is to eat protein first when they sit down to eat. Patients need to select what type of food they are eating first because they may not get to everything on a plate since they have a small stomach capacity. If the patient takes the required amount of protein, it will prevent the loss of muscle and the weight will come off the stored fat tissue in the body.

18. How many grams of protein should I eat?

This is a question that may have several answers since there is a great deal of disagreement even among nutritional experts. But in general if you consume 0.6 to 1.0 grams protein per kilogram of ideal body weight you will be eating a good amount. For more information on protein intake see the Post- operative Weight Loss Guide section of this book.

19. How soon after surgery will I resume taking my regular medications?

After discharge, you'll be able to resume your own medications. You won't be able to take two or more medications at the same time, so we will advise you to spread out medications at least 45 minutes to an hour apart. We do allow gel caps or capsules to be taken whole since they have the enteric coating and release the medication once they are in the stomach. Solid pills that are bigger than a plain M&M candy are better tolerated if they are crushed or split in half. If they are smaller than this size, you can take your medication whole.

20. What are typical discharge instructions?

Prior to discharge, your surgeon or someone from his or her team will go over certain information that is very important for you to follow. For example, in our case, we go over the discharge package, which includes paperwork, prescription, and the medications (which are given to you). I also go over extremely important routines you will be following over the next weeks: diet, physical activity and exercise, wound care, etc. It is important for you to ask any questions or express any doubts that you may have prior to going home. I advise you to write your questions down to avoid forgetting them and clarify them before leaving.

21. How will I have to eat immediately post-op and down the road?

Remember that the food ladder is clear liquids first, then full liquids, progressing afterwards to soft food and then regular food. For more information on this subject, I recommend you read the Postoperative Guide in this book.

22. Will I have problems with diarrhea post-op?

This depends on the patient. Some people will not have any changes in bowel movements, but others may experience loose stools. It is actually not diarrhea, it is loose stools because patients are only ingesting liquids. If no solids go in.. . no solids come out. If it gets too uncomfortable, contact your doctor's office for some advice.

23. What is the most important aspect of my post-op care?

The most important thing is following your post-op diet. This will ensure that your sleeve heals in an optimal way.

24. Should I expect to regain any of the lost weight?

As with any bariatric procedure, there is a chance you can regain weight if you don't follow the guidelines. If you follow them, the procedure will work for you and will keep the weight off permanently.

25. Will there be medications that I can no longer take post- op, or medications I won't absorb normally?

Once your stomach is healed, you will be able to take practically any medication you were taking prior to surgery although we don't recommend Non-Steroid Anti -Inflammatory (NSAID) medications like ibuprofen, naproxen, etc., since they are very irritating to the stomach's mucosa. If you have any doubts, please go over your medications you normally take with your surgeon to determine the optimal time to restart them and how to take them.

26. Will I get "sick" eating carbohydrates (sugars) or from eating fatty foods?

Typically, patients will not feel any different eating these types of food, since the only things altered with the gastric sleeve surgery are reducing the stomach's capacity and decreasing the patient's appetite. The dumping syndrome is commonly seen in patients who undergo a gastric bypass surgery. With this condition, patients develop elevated heart beat, palpitations, weakness, sweating, and dizziness. This happens because ingested foods bypass the stomach too rapidly and enter the small intestine largely undigested. There has been reported a very small percentage of patients who undergo gastric sleeve surgery and may experience some of these symptoms while eating carbohydrates.

27. What percentage of calories and fat will my body absorb post-op?

Your body will absorb 100% since we don't touch the intestines and they are not re-routed as with the gastric bypass. In a simplified way of putting it, the stomach digests and the intestines absorb; therefore, patients normally don't have any nutrient deficiencies as with the gastric bypass or duodenal switch.

28. What types of exercise do you recommend and at what stage post-op?

Cardiovascular is extremely helpful at any point post-op. Remember not to overdo it the first couple of weeks since your sleeve is still swollen and you will not be able to ingest large amounts of fluids at a time . Avoid getting dehydrated. I recommend a combination of cardiovascular and weight lifting after a month and a half post-op.

Chapter 10

Stories from My Patient Files

Misty (From a LAP-BAND® to a Gastric Sleeve)

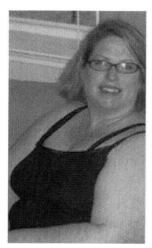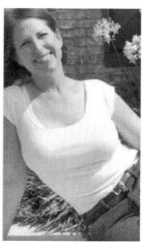

I absolutely love going shopping, trying on the latest fashionable styles in the dressing room, and with the exception of a few they always fit . . . and I look GOOD. There was a time in my not so distant past, for the span of most of my adult life, that this was not the case. Shopping was dreadful, dressing room mirrors had to be rigged as I tried to squeeze into a size 18 when a 20 would have been a better choice.

And bathing suits? Please! I didn't wear a bathing suit for an entire decade. It was depressing, and shopping forced me to see what was my truth . . . I was morbidly obese. My weight had fluctuated from a healthy weight of around 160 to a very unhealthy 280 lbs. I had clothes from a size 10 to a 22 . . . all in the same closet!!! Clothes that were a decade old sat patiently in the darkness of my deep closet waiting for me to FINALLY shed those pounds once and for all. I refused to let go of those old clothes collecting dust because in my rationale, if I tossed them out, then I was also tossing out any shred of hope left of finally beating the one battle in my life that I could not win . . . that of losing the weight and keeping it off.

I had gained and lost the same 45 lbs. a dozen times. I had done Weight Watchers® (4 different times, 3 different cities), Jenny Craig® (twice, 2 different states), Medifast® liquid diet (nearly put me in the hospital because I was so weak and dreadfully anemic), so many gym memberships I had lost count, and even a personal trainer that I never even met but paid in advance for 10 sessions because THIS was when I was FINALLY going to lose the weight and then it would MIRACULOUSLY never come back. I had pictures of actresses I had clipped from magazines that I would hope to motivate me to stop eating so much! I even purchased clothing in smaller sizes as motivation because I knew THIS time would be DIFFERENT . . . but it never was. My few thin members of my family and friends told me I just needed more willpower . . . that I wasn't trying HARD enough. I just needed to be stronger . . . I know now I was fighting my own evolutionary biology that had sustained my ancestors throughout times of famine, and my genetics won out. Twenty years went by with the same weight gain/weight loss with the same end result, and I reached a point in my life where I decided to take things to the next level. I was sick and tired . . . of being sick and tired.

Right before my 40th birthday, I made the decision to take action once and for all. I started researching weight loss surgery and I found Dr. Alvarez. I chose Dr. Alvarez for several reasons. One, my insurance company refused to pay for the surgery. I could be knocking on death's door, morbidly obese with a 100% guarantee that surgery would work, but my insurance company said "no way, will never happen, there is a written exclusion." Those executives who write these plans and crunch numbers all day in a tall downtown building didn't care how much of a fit I pitched or argued (usually these types of issues resolve for me because I am VERY persuasive and bug the crap out of them until they give in!) These fat cats in suits didn't budge. Since I was going to be have to be self-pay, surgery in my area was out of the question . . . I didn't have$15,000 + for the surgery, but surgery in Mexico was within my budget so I began researching. Dr. Alvarez had wonderful patient reviews I found online. Other patients had gone before me . . . they raved about how great he was, how thrilled they are, etc. Either he PAID all these people to say these things or just maybe . . . he was actually what they said he was . . . and I decided to find out for myself.

I called and left a message and HE called me back personally within an HOUR of leaving that message. He was polite, compassionate, and so very patient with my many questions. When I told my family and a select group of friends of my decision to have weight loss surgery . . . in MEXICO of all places, they thought I had for sure gone off the deep end and with absolute CERTAINTY would end up in the alleyway of some Mexican bar with only one kidney. I heard all the horror stories, how they reuse the surgical instruments without sterilization to save money. One of the best ones (besides the kidney in the alley story) that I was told was that the doctor would just give me a couple of incisions, and make it LOOK like I had surgery, but would take my money and bail, because so and so had an aunt's cousin's sister-in-law who had that done . . . none of which had any credibility or factual basis about the risks of surgery in Mexico.

Being the very stubborn, strong willed, independent and the Renegade I have always been, I went with my intuition, which had been pretty accurate up to that point and drove myself down from Dallas to Eagle Pass, Texas, to get the surgery. I admit to you readers that I was afraid because I had never met anyone who had surgery in Mexico personally. I had the LAP-BAND® from Dr. Alvarez on March15, 2007. Early that morning, Dr. A's cousin picked me up at my hotel in Eagle Pass to drive me across the border. When I met her, my first thought was . . . well she looks normal (Sorry Rosie!) I met Dr. Alvarez and was smitten with the very handsome young doctor with his infectious smile and charming nature. I met some ladies that were from Texas, two sisters and Mom, all who got the sleeve 2 days before and were getting ready for their trip home. One, a teacher, could sense my nervousness and came to pat me on the back and give me a pep talk. I felt better after talking to her, got changed into my hospital gown, and waited . . . After the procedural taking of blood, etc., they wheeled me to the operating room . . . the moment of truth had arrived and my strength and Renegade attitude started to wane and I began crying . . . I was so afraid. I gripped tightly to the photograph of my children encased in lamination that I brought for support and showed it to Dr. Alvarez before the Anesthesiologist put me under, as if to demonstrate my importance of being a mother to these three young kids . . . so please don't take my kidney and dump me in an alley . . . It was one of those profound moments in your life that you can remember frame by frame . . . he told me as he wiped the tears from my eyes. . . he said,

"Your tears are wasted here . . . save them for something more important because you are going to be just fine." I woke up in my hospital room a couple of hours later and got up immediately to walk around. It was really that easy. Surgery and I typically do not get along well. The anesthesia causes horrible nausea and vomiting, but I had neither of those for the first surgery in my life. I drove myself back home the next day to Dallas and started my liquid diet.

After about 6 weeks, I got my first band fill. Finding a doctor in Dallas that would fill a band placed in Mexico was actually very easy as there are several doctors more than willing to do it. At $200 for 5 minutes of actual work of filling the band, it was a goldmine for a few smart doctors. I lost around80 lbs with the band but not without significant problems caused by severe acid reflux and getting food stuck. I was adamant to get the weight off, so I suffered through the inconvenience and discomfort. It became such a hassle and the list of foods that I could not eat was growing longer than the foods that I could eat. The inconsistency from one day to the next was baffling . . . One day I would have good restriction and only eat small amounts, and other days, around PMS time of the month, the band seemed wide open and I could eat like I could prior to getting the band placed. Then as quickly as it came on, it would have so much restriction that I could only drink water. By the time I paid over $2,000 for fills and unfills over almost a year, the difference in the band vs. the sleeve would have paid for itself. This was a very expensive lesson for me.

The acid reflux and constant vomiting caused me to seek out a gastroenterologist for help. Sleepless nights of sitting up in a chair because acid shoots up in your throat and you have to jump up and spit it out was taking a toll on my quality of life. If I have less fluid in the band, then I don't lose weight and keep it off. So I suffered until I got the results of an endoscope. I found I had damaged my esophagus to the point that it was called Barrett's Esophagus, a precancerous condition. I contacted Dr. Alvarez and after consulting with him, decided to have the band removed and replaced with the VSG sleeve.

On Thanksgiving Day, 2008, I had the sleeve done with Dr. Alvarez again in Mexico. Having been through the drill before, I wasn't afraid at all. I knew I was in good hands, having referred family and friends to Dr. Alvarez during the year I had lost the weight. After 2 routine nights in the hospital, I came back to Dallas and after a few weeks of the required liquid diet, resumed my life but THIS time it was permanent, and I had no foods on my list of unpermitted foods. I could eat all the salad, asparagus, bread, pasta, but this time I had the sleeve a.k.a. "Food Police" that tells you when you have had enough.

Two years have passed since getting the sleeve. I maintain a very healthy weight for my height of 5'11", between 165-172 lbs. and wear a comfortable size 10. Maintaining my weight has been so easy. If I feel my jeans feeling a little snug, I just cut back on my carbohydrate intake, focus on eating my protein and veggies, and I stay at a comfortable size. It has really been that effortless compared to the yo-yo dieting effect of half of my life. My only regret was not getting the sleeve in the first place, Dr. Alvarez tried to tell me before getting banded but the difference of several thousand dollars was more important at the time than listening to him. I paid equal that amount with all the fills/unfills I had that first year.

I am so thankful, that as I enter the second half of my life, I can focus on living instead of trying to lose weight and dreaming of all the things I could be doing if I weren't so overweight. Food will always be my drug of choice and primary coping mechanism (I am working on this!!), but with the sleeve in place, I can eat a few Hershey kisses and get the same satisfaction as a giant 1 lb. Hershey bar would have pre-weight loss surgery. It's the best investment you can give yourself because your quality of life can't have a price tag put on it. The money I save on food I now spend on shopping for skinny jeans and bikinis . . . and the mirror in the dressing room just loves me. That gorgeous lady smiles every time I go to try clothes on and I am so thrilled to only have ONE size of clothing in my closet . . . Thank you, Dr. Alvarez, for providing me with the support these last few years and for becoming a friend as well as a doctor. . . .

Susan

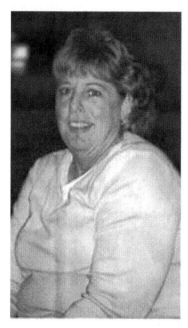 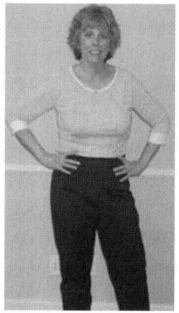

I have been overweight the majority of my life and have lost and gained hundreds of pounds in my quest for thinness. It never got so out of hand as when I looked at my photo from my birthday gathering in March 2005. When my co-worker sent the pictures she had taken of me I just cried. I thought I looked OK, but looking at this person in the photos, I didn't even recognize myself. What happened, was all I could ask myself.

Thus began my search for something to take care of my

obesity. I knew a gal who had done the LAP-BAND®
locally, so I picked her brain a little bit and had
watched her transformation, so I decided that this
might be the key to my own weight loss success. In the
States, my insurance wouldn't cover this since my BMI
didn't meet criteria . . . even the doctor I met with told
me to gain another 80 pounds then come back and see
him. Are you crazy? So, in May 2005, I set off for
Monterrey Mexico, alone and had the LAP -BAND®
procedure done. Of course, standard verbiage going
through my head once home was "what have you
done?" and "you did it where?" Needless to say, my
next 1 yr with the band was not what I had hoped and
wasn't without its regret and frustration. I had to go
out of town to even find someone willing to do my fills,
even went back to Mexico to have one done. The truly
sad part of the whole ordeal was despite doing
everything right, I only lost 35 pounds, wound up with
a port infection that almost killed me, and had to have
the stupid thing totally removed. However, that was
the best thing that could have happened to me. In the
interim of healing from this and of course gaining back
that 35 pounds I had worked so hard to lose, I
subsequently had the VSG performed and the rest,

shall we say, is history. My recovery was so easy, I lost my 70 pounds in 8-9months, never had a lick of trouble, and it has truly been the best thing that has ever happened to me. September 2010 will be my 4th year anniversary and it has been an incredible journey. I know I have conquered my obesity problem, have discovered I now really like who I see in the mirror, and wouldn't change a thing . . . well, except to have never done the band in the first place. The most incredible thing to come out of this whole ordeal is the fact I have the privilege of now working for this truly talented surgeon who cares about his work. Helping others is his passion and it shows. I have met so many wonderful patients along my own road and will be forever grateful.

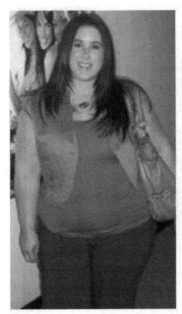
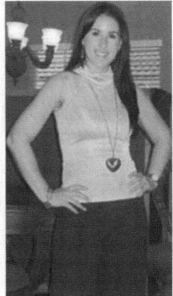

Amy

I never had a problem with my weight until after I had my child and became a stay at home mom, my activity level dropped and so did my discipline for dieting.

I had tried anything and everything including senseless diets, diet pills, etc. . . . However, it was always just a quick fix, I would eventually go back to my starting weight and would put on even more weight than when I began. All that yo-yo dieting just made me balloon up to 235lbs. When I got so heavy that my back and feet were in constant pain and I was just tired of all the senseless diets and suffering, that's when I began to look into bigger and better options. I ran across a website which offered a forum with weight loss patients that would share their stories.

I researched all the different weight loss surgeries there were out there and I decided the gastric sleeve was the right type of weight loss surgery I wanted. I began to post questions on the forum and made some great post-sleeve surgery friends who guided me to Dr. Alvarez.

It took me and my family a while to get over the whole idea of traveling to Mexico to get such a big surgery.

However, after a year of research and talking to Dr. Alvarez and getting to know him and his patients I was 100% confident in the surgery and the doctor.

Dr. Alvarez's coordinator Susan, who is also a patient of Dr. Alvarez, was there for me every step of the way to answer all my questions and make me feel excited about what I was about to do.

When I met Dr. Alvarez I felt so comfortable I just knew I would be in good hands; he took his time with me and was completely honest with me. I never felt lost or confused. Both Dr. Alvarez and Susan had prepared me to what was going to happen every step of the way.

Now I'm happy to write that it has been 3 years post-surgery and I have lost a total of 100 lbs. I look and feel like a new woman. I'm so grateful for the sleeve, for Dr. Alvarez, and his wonderful team.

The best part of this is that I still keep in contact with Dr. Alvarez and Susan and I'm even thinking of going back soon and getting my gallstones removed with the best surgeon I know: Dr. Alvarez.

Kathryn

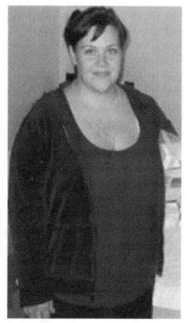 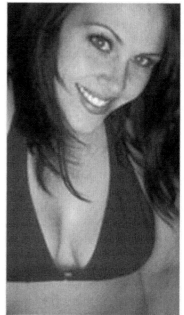

My psychological battle with obesity started in my childhood. I was always a thin little girl with big knobby knees; this was mostly due to the fact that I often went without food and was almost always hungry. A single mother of 7 children who was too proud to accept a handout raised me. Oftentimes we would share one burger between the eight of us, being told not to be a pig, take a bite, and pass it on. Sometimes the one meal a day that was provided came from our local homeless shelter. One year they gave away boxes of food for Thanksgiving; that year was one of the years we were homeless. We lived in a tent and the shelter had no way of knowing that an uncooked turkey and boxed food could not feed kids living with nowhere to cook it. As I grew older I learned to fend for myself, asking high school friends for the rest of their fries, a drink of their soda or the other half of their candy bar. When I got my first job at 15 it happen to be in a Las Vegas casino gift shop. There, I had access to food. All the soda, candy, and beef jerky I was hungry enough to steal. Every once in a while I would get desperate enough and take $5 from the cash register to buy a sandwich or something more substantial and hope to put it back on payday. Life started to get a little better when I brought home money that my mother would spend on groceries. I quickly figured out that obtaining means was a way out of hunger. I soon got married, had a child, and went on to get a college degree (yes, in that order). By the time I was 20, I owned my own home and had made a wonderful life for myself. The happier life got, the bigger I became. To me, happiness meant being able to eat when I wanted. I ate to treat myself after a long day, I ate to deal with the stresses of motherhood, I ate simply because I COULD. One day, my husband, our boys, and myself were vacationing in a California theme park. My knees hurt, I was out of breath, and I was worried I might not fit on the next ride. I was 27 years old, I was 5'3", 232 pounds, a size 22, and I would have had a better time if we could have sat at the restaurant eating our way through the day. I knew something had to change. I could no longer use food to reward myself. It was killing me and actually robbing me of the wonderful things I had worked so hard for. That night I went on an Internet search looking for a way to fix myself. I came across Obesityhelp.com. I read the stories for hours and cried as I looked over before and after photos. One name kept coming up: Dr. Guillermo Alvarez. I read all about him and the sleeve procedure he was performing. I saw the amazing transformation in his clients and wanted it for myself. I saw the happiness that this doctor and his staff were providing for thousands, and after a few weeks of research I had no doubts that this was it for me. I called and got to talk with Susan; she quickly set up everything I needed to start a happier and healthier life. On May 15, 2008, I was in a Mexican operating room with the highly skilled surgeon Dr. Alvarez having a gastric sleeve procedure performed. That was two and a half years ago now and it is hard to believe it actually came to fruition.

I am now 29 years old. I weigh 120lbs. and am a rocking size 4. Unless I tell them, no one would ever know that I have had weight-loss surgery (even after I tell them few people can hardly believe it). I no longer struggle with food. Dr. Alvarez has provided me with a wonderful gift that I know has not only added quality, but has added years to my life. There are few words to describe the degree of hope that Dr. Alvarez and the sleeve give people struggling with obesity. The best way for me to say it is this: He gives life. I thank him for that every day.

John

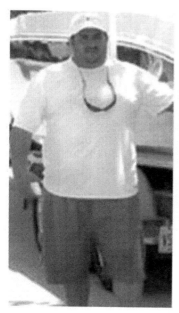 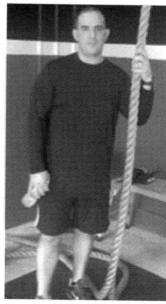

Well, what can I say about the VSG? This has been by far the most important decision of my life. It has truly been life changing for me in a very positive manner. As a child, I was always in good shape and was never a fat kid. Always performed at the top levels in all sports as well as competed in karate most of my life from the age of 4 till about 29 years of age. After I decreased my high level of fitness, being married and raising a family and work and so forth, I slowly started adding the pounds. Between 10-15 lbs. per year as if it were very little weight to add; after 6-8 years of that rhythm, I ended up very heavy and unhealthy, uncomfortable for a long time. The bigger I got, the more sugars I craved and the worse the eating habits became. To add to the equation, becoming obese not only added weight and unhealthy risk factors, but also a great deal of stress and depression associated with unhappiness and lack of self-esteem. The yoyo diets went on for years, some more successful than others, but in the end, I always managed to pileup the weight with a few more pounds added every time. Before turning forty, I decided to look into weight loss surgery and looked into various options available at the time in the market. I did extensive research worldwide on the latest and most innovative procedures with the safest results and most significant success and ended up deciding to go with the VSG procedure, finding this to be the most appropriate for me at the time and having found Dr. Alvarez to be the leading authority in the world with the most amount of cases performed of this procedure. I felt comfortable enough to travel to his location and get treated by him. It was truly an amazing experience. Hands down the most courteous, professional, and best bedside manners I have yet to experience. It truly felt like a lifelong friend taking care of me. Not to mention a pain free surgery from day one and on. It was truly a blessing, and after losing over 100 lbs, which I did within 9 months, it was truly a remarkable comeback in my life. Thanks to Dr. Alvarez and his complete staff, I have regained what I thought was lost at one point in my life: my health, my intense level of fitness, my desire for living, my vitality in all areas, my self-esteem, and, most important, a quality of life that will allow me to grow older in a much healthier fashion. My eating habits are much more conscious and healthier, and my appetite has been pretty much stable and rational. It has truly made a huge difference in my life, as well as the lives of all of those who surround me. From 300 lbs. to around 188 in less than a year, and I have kept it off and steady without any major sacrifice. Although I do exercise quite a bit a few times a week at a pretty intense level. My life was slow before, now life is good once again. Thank you, Dr. Alvarez. You are truly a lifesaver.

Betsy

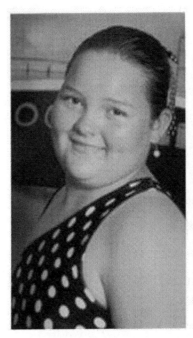
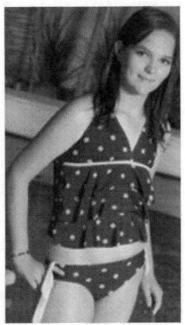

I had weight problems since I was little, but it was when I was11 that I asked my parents to help me find a good option for weight loss. I knew about the surgery options because my uncle (Dr. Alvarez) does that, and so I told my parents I wanted that. I really wanted to be thin, like my friends. I wanted to look and feel good. As a part of my process, my parents took me to a psychologist, because it was important to know if surgery was an answer for me, since I had already tried every other possible option without any results. So the psychologist told my parents she believed it was a great option for me, that I was mentally ready for it and that I really needed something to help my self-esteem, to grow up being more confident. When I turned 14, I had the gastric sleeve. When I woke up after the surgery I remember having some stomachache; my uncle told me it was from the gas they use to do the surgery, so they gave me something and it went away. I remember the next day I was feeling good, I had no pain whatsoever, I was getting out of bed and moving without any help. I stayed one night in the hospital and then my uncle let me go home. I had to do a special diet my uncle gave me for 3 weeks. It wasn't easy, but I wasn't hungry, and that helped. When the 3 weeks passed, I started eating little by little everything I used to eat, but much less. There are some things I almost don't eat anymore, like soda. I don't like the way it feels when I drink it; I prefer water now. My picture is from 9 months after the surgery. I had already reached my goal weight. I feel great. Now I like doing some things I didn't enjoy before, like shopping for clothes! I feel pretty and I now like it when people look at me. I'm in dance lessons, and I love swimming too. I think the surgery is a very good option for people my age, because it makes you feel and look good, which is very important. I'm very happy I finally did it. It changed my life.

For More Stories Just Like These

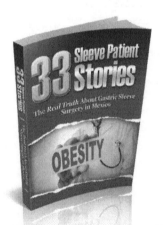

Get a *FREE Copy* of 33 Gastric Sleeve Stories From My Patient Files

Go to www.SleeveStories.com

Made in the USA
San Bernardino, CA
14 March 2018